AN UNDERVIEW
OF MENTAL ILLNESS

An Underview
of Mental Illness

Michael Crawford
"Bipolar II"

Writer's Showcase
presented by *Writer's Digest*
San Jose New York Lincoln Shanghai

An Underview of Mental Illness

Writer's Showcase
presented by *Writer's Digest*
an imprint of iUniverse.com, Inc.

For information address:
iUniverse.com, Inc.
5220 S 16th, Ste. 200
Lincoln, NE 68512
www.iuniverse.com

ISBN: 0-595-14107-2

Printed in the United States of America

For My Children

Epigraph

"Everyone can master a grief but he that has it."

William Shakespeare
Much Ado About Nothing, 3.2, 27

Contents

Preface

Having spent fourteen years as an improperly medicated "manic-depressive", then five as a properly medicated "bipolar II", I have seen a small part of the mental health industry from the bottom up. Some of the things I have learned are:

There are serious mental illnesses, mental disorders and behavioral disorders.

Yes, serious mental illnesses run in families, but their eruption is not a sure thing. Many things must align just so before one flowers. It is not preordained fate that the children and grandchildren of the seriously mentally ill will follow suit.

Substantial, fabulous progress has been made in explaining the eruption of the serious affective mental illnesses and in containing them; but no cure for any of them has yet been found and none may ever be.

Every case of mental illness is slightly different because of each of us has unique chemistry and unique experiences. Therefore, finding the right combination of drugs and therapy for each mentally ill person is a trial and error process.

In my nineteen years of experience as a bipolar II, I have found our Nation's safety net to be slow, frustrating, perplexing and effective. The Veteran's Administration provided all my health care needs when I had no resources at all. The Louisiana Rehabilitation Services re-trained me for a job that I can perform. And Social Security Disability Income has been as effective as any drug that I have taken for my illness. Yet, I received generously from the safety net because I know how to ask for help…and that nags me. I worry a lot about the lost souls who are not veterans and who don't know how to ask.

Acknowledgements

It is said that when a person is ready to learn, a teacher will appear. Eve Struve, Ph.D., has been mine.

1

The Brain vs. the Mind

History

Mental illness has always been part of the human experience. Prior to 1751, when the first "therapeutic" hospitals (for the wealthy) were opened in Europe, the mentally ill were treated with punishment, confinement, torture, surgery, straightjackets, pity, contempt, and ridicule. Peasant families in Europe sometimes kept their "mad" members in holes, not only to reduce care to a minimum, but also to hide the family's shame. Many such attitudes survive today, greatly baffling the mentally ill as they try to find their way in societies that worship perfect people.

Yet, even as societies despise their mentally ill, they rush to embrace a few of them as "Great Leaders". Hitler, Stalin, Idi Amin, Pol Pot, Saddam Hussien, and Slobidan Milosevic are a short list of such leaders in the Twentieth Century–a contradiction that brings to mind Bob Dylan's wonderful lyric, "steal a little and they call you 'thief', steal a lot and they call you 'king'".

The application of real science to mental illness began in 1861, when the microscope made it possible for Wilhelm Griesinger, a German neurologist, to declare the condition to be, in function, an illness of nerves and brain.

The conceptual breakthrough for classifying mental illnesses came from another German neurologist, Emil Kraepelin. Unable to use a microscope because of poor eyesight, Kraepelin resorted to precise record keeping of the patients in the mental institution that he ran. On vacation, one day, he decided to sort his hundreds of records by prognosis (that is, by prospect of recovery). In one group there was clearly no prospect of recovery. That group contained the true schizophrenics. In a second group, he discovered a class of patients that mysteriously got well, left the hospital for a period of time, only to return worse off than before. Kraepelin named the illness of that second group, who had previously been thought to be schizophrenic, "Manic-Depression" (now called "Bipolar Illness Disorder"). The third group was characterized more by "badness", than by "madness" and they eventually became what we call today the behavioral/personality disorders.[1]

Note the progression of refinement. With Griesinger, the Function Neurologist, "Madness" became "nerve illness". With Kraepelin, the Classification Neurologist, nerve illness became "schizophrenia", "manic-depression", and (eventually) "behavioral disorders".

Then came the Freudian revolution with concepts so powerful that it claimed our understanding of mental illness for six decades. Sigmund Freud, too, was trained as a neurologist, and he never totally strayed from Griesinger's fundamental concept of mental illness as a nerve illness. Beguiled, however, by the ability of hypnosis to release the hidden remembrances of the "Mind", (analogous to a computer suddenly remembering software forgotten "on purpose"), Freud created a new "Mind Science" (my term) which he named "Psychoanalysis".

Based upon guided talk, which yielded "free association" of conscious thoughts with unconscious memories (and the unseen hand of childhood sexuality) the new approach to mental illness became, by the 1940's, the dominant mental illness treatment in Europe. Twenty years

---

1   Wender, P.H. & Klein, D.F., (1981), *Mind, Mood, and Medicine.* New York, N.Y., Farrar, Straus, Giroux.

later, in the 1960's, psychoanalysis became the dominant mental illness treatment in America.[2]

The limitations of Psychoanalysis are, however, great. By his own admission, Freud's methods could do nothing for schizophrenics or psychotics, such as manics.

The Biopsychiatric Revolution

Beguiling and endlessly fascinating, much of Freud's "Mind Science" did not survive the test of time. Instead, "Brain Science" overtook Mind Science in 1949, when the manic-calming properties of *lithium carbonate* were discovered. In 1950, the brain chemical, *serotonin*, was identified with depression. Also in the 1950's, electroconvulsive therapy (ECT) for severe depression was found to produce results. In 1954 *Thorazine* was approved for use with schizophrenics. *Thorazine* calmed schizophrenics so well that state governments, wishfully thinking that their wards had become normal, began "de-institutionalizing" them. But the states didn't understand that mental illness is almost invisible to those who have it–almost all of us mentally ill begin our illnesses "thinking" that we are perfectly normal. Once the schizophrenics were free of their supervised care, they stopped taking their medicine. Many of them now live on our streets like rabbits among dogs. Indeed, if our civilization is judged by how well we care for the least among us, we aren't one.

In 1955, *Miltown* was approved, and the "tranquilizer era" began. In 1958, the first antidepressive, *Tofranic* was approved. In 1987, the breakthrough antidepressant *Prozac* was approved to great fanfare. Called "The happiness pill" and the subject of endless jokes, such as a morose man finding "The Bluebird of *Prozac*" sitting on his widow sill, this breakthrough drug revolutionized the treatment of depression because

---

2   Shorter, E., (1997). *A History of Psychiatry*, New York, NY: John Wiley & Sons, Inc.

it is very effective with very few side effects. The same may be said for the other two members of the *Prozac* family, *Paxil* and *Zoloft*–with the reservation that every human has different chemistry and, thus, different reactions to drugs. Just as there is no "one size fits all" drug for mania, there is no "one size fits all" antidepressant. *Paxil*, for example, is a miracle drug for me; but *Zoloft* makes me want to curl up like a fetus and *Prozac* makes me cry.

The effectiveness of *Prozac* caused many in the mental health field to ask, "If a drug can diminish depression so effectively, how can depression be, as Freud defined it, 'anger turned inward'"? The answer is that 'anger turned inward' is still a possible explanation for the eruption of *exogenous depression* (that is, "situational depression" caused by life events); but modern drugs can contain all forms of depression, including *indigenous depression* (the kind produced not by life events, but by faulty brain chemistry).

Can it, therefore, once again be said that mental illness is an illness of the nerves and brain alone? No, not yet. Perhaps never. First of all, there are many complex, interlocking, chemical and electrical systems, such as gene expression, secondary messengers and the endocrine system, which make defining the boundaries of the "brain" and "mind" very difficult. In addition, there are the parasympathetic and sympathetic systems, which connects the brain with the eyes, salivation, lungs, heart, bowels, liver, bladder and rectum (among other things). The greatest reason, however, is that the most human characteristic of all, memory, has yet to be explained; thus, memory itself, at least for now, belongs in the wispy category, "Mind".

Consider these things:

(1) Brain/minds change over time. There are two organizing concepts to explain brain/mind change, namely "plasticity" and "engrams". "Plasticity" is the ability of the human brain/mind to be flexible in learning and in modifying previously stored learning, thus changing its state

of being continuously and forever. An "engram" is a hypothetical change in a neuron postulated to account for the persistence of memory.

(2) The brain/mind has never been, as once thought, a black box like a computer, wired permanently by age two or three. Rather, it is now recognized to be a lifelong learning "machine", not unlike a vacuum cleaner that sucks up everything in its path.

(3) In an ideal state of plasticity, the brain/mind remodels itself constantly in response to constantly incoming experiences: aging, hormone changes, illnesses, injuries, learning and environment.

(4) In a faulty state of plasticity, the brain/mind can stop remodeling itself. "Phantom pain", where an amputated limb once existed, is an example of such faulty plasticity. Obsessive-compulsive disorder might be another.

(5) In a hypothetical state of total plasticity, the brain/mind could forget its memories and begin reorganizing continuously.[3]

Faulty plasticity is an intriguing hypothesis for bipolar eruption and persistence. As someone who has lived within the illness for nineteen years, I intuitively dig this proposed explanation. It seems to explain why, when I was improperly medicated and chaotic in my bipolar disorder, I kept confusing the past with the present.

Here is an example: I had just left my first psychiatric hospital. I was on *lithium carbonate* (it was the only drug available to me at the time) and was counseling weekly with a psychiatrist. I found a job as the General Manager of a small manufacturing plant. (It is not rare for Bipolars to get good jobs. While in mania, they can do almost anything. Because of their unstable emotions, however, holding good jobs is another matter entirely.) Our uniform vendor supplied the soap for our washrooms. I noticed that we were out of soap for a day or two. I called and asked that soap be sent out at once. Nothing happened. I noticed

---

3   *http://www.washingtonpost.com/wp-srv/health/daily/sept99/brain28.htm*

that the workers were eating their lunches with grimy hands. I exploded with a volcanic anger that was way out of proportion to the situation. Had my emotions been normal, I would probably have solved the problem by buying soap at a food store. But no, I did nothing reasonable. I called the uniform vendor and fired them, then called a new vendor and had soap in the washrooms within hours. As the anger subsided, another long and deep depression began.

Later in the week, I discussed the incident and its depression with my counselor. With her assistance, I dredged up the following memory from my early teens. I was sitting on the back steps with my father. He was dressed to go to a wedding. My mother opened the back door and said, in her Other Voice (i.e., her long-suffering one),

"Everidge, make sure your finger-nails are clean."

"They will be."

"Well, I don't want to be seen with you if they aren't."

Dad looked at his well-worn hands, which had fingernails black with tungsten-carbide dust, the material that, with his labor, supported us all. He looked at me and said, softly,

"How does she expect me to earn a living without getting my hands dirty?"

Recalling that fingernail memory from my teens, and the range of emotions that I felt over my father's humiliation, from sympathy to anger, was the first of many instances in which I would make a connection between my childhood experiences and their adult expressions. At the time, though, I was not as fascinated by the process as I am now. Rather, I was flabbergasted. I had stored an old memory, and its anger, for thirty or so years, until a current event roughly aligned with it; then out it poured, its anger as fresh as the day it was born.

Or, in my understanding of behavioral neurology, the engrams of a teenage experience were recalled in the process of storing a roughly-similar adult experience in short-term memory.

The Amygdala

The hypothetical culprit in the bipolar disorder faulty-memory hypothesis is the amygdala, which some medical students call "Amy". The amygdala is known to be the most easily kindled part of the limbic system (that is, "kindled" into starting epilepsy and, perhaps, bipolar eruptions).[4] Furthermore, it is generally agreed that the amygdala is involved in short-term memory storage, and in determining the location of such storage.[5] The most important concept in the amygdala's relationship to the bipolar disorder faulty-memory hypothesis, however, is the strong suspicion that most memories include an affective or emotional component.[6] Thus, bipolar disorder may result from a faulty amygdala storing highly emotional memories in a faulty way. Such highly emotional memories might then be recalled by a faulty amygdala, in a faulty process, when any emotion similar to, but not exactly right with any current situation. A simple example of such a process would be a bipolar disorder twin who lost her sister to suicide. Any mention of suicide, no matter how remote from her, brings the memory of her dying sister erupting back into her current memory as if it were a present, not a past event.

It must be remembered, however, that proving this hypothesis, or any other in brain/mind science, is extraordinarily complex. There are over 12,000 *billion* neurons (cells) in the human nervous system, 10,000 billion of them in the brain. Each one of the little rascals participates in all the forms of conscious and unconscious experiences. This

---

4   Goddard, G.V.; McIntyre, D.C. & Leech, C.K. (1969). A permanent change in brain function resulting from daily electrical stimulation. *Experimental Neurology* 25: 295-330.

5   McGaugh, J. L.; Bermudez-Rattoni, F.; Prado-Alcala, R. A., (1995). *Plasticity In The Central Nervous System*. Lawrence Erlbaum Associates, Publishers, Mahwah, New Jersey, p. 34

6   Izquierdo,(1995). *Plasticity In The Central Nervous System*, Lawrence Erlbaum Associates, Publishers, Mahwah, New Jersey. p. 51

is a fantastically huge number that is far greater than the number of stars in our galaxy, which makes exploring our inner universe is every bit as complicated as exploring the outer one. In fact, scientists have probably gone further in exploring and explaining outer space than inner space. In outer space, we know the functions of planets, moons, comets, asteroids, pulsars, photons, brown stars, white stars, blue stars, red stars, novae, and so on. In inner space, scientists aren't absolutely sure of the function of anything because all neurons seem to be connected to all others. Not only that, neurons communicate with each other by both electricity and chemicals.

Even so, just as it can be said that human bodies obviously create hunger, it can also be said that human brain/minds obviously create learning and memory. And anyone who has studied mentally ill people can tell you that faulty learning and confused memory are primary characteristics of serious mental illness.

A major breakthrough in brain/mind science occurred in 1969. That was the year when Drs. G. V. Goddard, D.C. McIntyre and C.K. Leech published their paper called, "A permanent change in brain function resulting from daily electrical stimulation".[7] It described the process by which they induced epilepsy in the brains of rats by implanting electrodes in their limbic systems. The mere inducement of epilepsy, however, was not the real "shocker"–that stunning discovery came later, when, after repeated electrical stimulation, the rats "learned and memorized" epilepsy and no longer needed electrical stimulation to go into seizures. Goddard and his team named the process "the kindling effect" because, like kindling wood in a fireplace, a small amount of electricity applied to a certain spot in the limbic system produced a larger "fire" that eventually became self-sustaining. That "certain spot"

---

7   Goddard, G.V.; McIntyre, D.C. & Leech, C.K. (1969). A permanent change in brain function resulting from daily electrical stimulation. *Experimental Neurology* 25: 295-330.

was the amygdala, the brain structure long postulated to regulate certain emotional functions in humans, such as anger, fear, happiness and sexual stimulation.

The Peerless Dr. Post

Dr. R.M. Post, a psychiatrist, is the Head of the Biological Psychiatric Branch of the National Institute of Mental Health. He and his colleagues at the NIMH have developed a variation on the Goddard electrical kindling effect that they call "The Kindling Model of Affective Illness". More than anything else that I have encountered in my nineteen years as a bipolar, the Post "Kindling model" explains to my satisfaction what happened to me in 1981 and after. Here is my version of his research.

Since the work of Kraepelin, four characteristics of bipolar disorder have been known. It has (1) more than one distinct form; (2) tremendous variability in its clinical course; (3) a pattern of cycle acceleration; (4) progression from precipitated to autonomous episodes. Of these observations by Kraepelin, Post writes,

> Since 1921, "[Kraepelin's] clinical observations have been documented and re-documented in more formal clinical studies. In systematic studies examining the issue of cycle acceleration, the general pattern of decreasing duration of well intervals as a function of successive episodes has been supported in virtually every study."[8]

Missing from Kraepelin's work, however, is an explanation of how the illness starts. That is why Post became interested in Goddard's kindling effect. If small amounts of electricity administered to a rat's

---

8   Post, R.M. & Weiss, S. B., (1995). F.E. Bloom (Ed.), & D.J. Kupfer (Ed.), *Psychopharmacology: The Forth Generation of Progress.* (pp 1155-69). Raven Press,. Ltd., New York. **See Book**

amygdala can "start" epilepsy, Post asked, could a similar sort of thing start bipolar disorder in humans?

So far, Post answers this question with an unequivocal "perhaps"–for the same reason mentioned earlier, namely that deciding anything about a human brain with 10,000 billion neurons is extraordinarily difficult. He does argue, however, that in at least some patients, bipolar disorder eruption and evolution mimics Goddard's kindling effect in that stress replaces electricity as the stimulant, and that once stimulated, the illness follows the course known since Kraepelin…

Post's model is, in the scientific method, a hypothesis awaiting confirmation by other scientists in other laboratories, hospitals and clinics. This confirmation process has begun. Ghaemi, et.al.[9] reviewed the results of twelve studies of 2,578 total bipolar disorder patients. All of the studies tested two predictions of the kindling model: That psychological blows would occur frequently in the early course of the illness, and that frequency of fully fledged bipolar disorder episodes would increase in the later course of the illness. Eight of the twelve studies confirmed these two predictions, pretty good support for a hypothesis.

So is the fact that other mental illnesses, such as panic attacks, compulsive rituals and post traumatic stress disorder (PTSD) and even migraine headaches can be shown to mimic the kindling genesis of epilepsy and bipolar disorder, although they do not manifest in the same way.[10] Because they don't, it is important to emphasize how Post's Kindling *model* differs from that of Goddard's *effect*. Consider, first, what the Post kindling model is not.

---

9   Ghaemi, S.N.; Boiman, E.E.; Goodwin, F.K. (1999). Kindling and second messengers: an approach to the neurobiology of recurrence in bipolar disorder. *Biological Psychiatry, 45 (2)*: 137-44.

10   Post, R.M. & Weiss, S.R.B. (1998), Sensitization and Kindling Phenomena in Mood, Anxiety, and Obsessive-Compulsive Disorders: The Role of Serotonergic Mechanisms in Illness Progression. *Biological Psychiatry, 44*: 193-206.

First, Goddard's kindling effect models epilepsy, the end product of which is seizures. Post's kindling model models bipolar disorder, the end product of which is unstable moods, which are not likely be caused by seizures. Secondly, electrical stimulation, which produces epilepsy in Goddard's kindling effect, does not produce bipolar disorder. Thirdly, the brain circuits involved in epilepsy do not appear to be the same as those involved in bipolar disorder. Finally, there is not an exact match between the ways that identical drugs work in epilepsy and bipolar disorder. Therefore, Post's kindling model does not replicate Goddard's kindling effect in any measurable way. There are, however, similarities, shown in **bold** below:

	Goddard's "Effect"	*Post's "Model"*
Major brain involvement:	**Amygdala**	**Amygdala**
Stimulant to brain:	Electricity	Psychological blow(s)
Response of brain:	Epilepsy	Bipolar disorder
Progressive increase in illness severity?	**Yes**	**Yes**
Intermittent reinforcement yields spontaneous episodes?	**Yes**	**Yes**
Process mimics learning?	**Yes**	**Yes**
Containment with similar drugs?	**Yes**	**Yes**

So, there are differences and similarities in Goddard's Kindling and in Post's Model. To me, a non-scientist, the similarities are greater than the differences; but good science is always careful science, and it is definitely careful to emphasize the differences.

Dr. Post and his colleagues began to publish their kindling model discoveries in 1982.[11] Here is my summary of their research and discoveries, published over the next eighteen years.

1. The illness has a strong genetic component.

2. Childhood and adolescent traumas proceed bipolar disorder eruptions and "train" neuronal pathways in the brain/mind for later illness-inducing stress.

3. A first eruption of bipolar disorder, or "kindling", succeeds or fails in direct relationship to the quality of previous traumatic memories and neuronal pathway training. Thus, childhood and adolescent traumas are the parents of bipolar disorder eruption.

4. A kindling event alone will not flame into self-sustaining bipolar disorder. For that to happen, a kindling event must be subsequently reinforced in an intermittent way in accordance with the discoveries of behavioral psychologists such as Pavlov, Watson, Thorndike and Skinner.

5. Lacking intervention with drug and counseling therapies, bipolar disorder eruption graduates from a psychosocial reaction stage (with reinforcement) into a stage of internal genesis in which "episodes beget episodes". At this point, the illness becomes automatic and uncontrollable.

6. In its advanced stage, even if stabilized with drug and counseling therapies, illness "personality" continues to evolve. Because kindling of bipolar disorder develop from genetic inheritance and environment (such as childhood traumas), all of which are unique to the afflicted, and because each psychosocial reinforcement sequence is unique to the

---

11 Post, R.M.; Uhde, T.W.; Putnam, F.W.; Ballenger, J.C.; and Berrettini, W.H. (1982). Kindlingand carbamazepine in affective illness. *The Journal of Nervous and Mental Disease*, 170,12: 17-731.

afflicted, each case of bipolar disorder manifests and evolves uniquely within these major (but not limited to) characteristics:

(1) A *few cycles* through a usual period consisting of these three stages, the order of which may differ from patient to patient:
    a. Mania.
    b. Well interval.
    c. Depression.

(2) *Rapid cycling* of more than four swings per year, such as (but not limited to):
    a. Cycling of all three stages
    b. Cycling of mania and depression with no well interval
    c. Intermittent appearance of the well interval
    d. More mania than depression
    e. More depression than mania

(3) *Chaotic cycles* from which there is limited relief.

7. As illness personality evolves, drugs that originally stabilized the illness require augmentation. That is, new drugs that restrain new personality manifestations are added to original courses without discontinuing original drugs.

There are also kindling-like mechanisms in other affective illnesses, such as "Post Traumatic Stress Syndrome", commonly called "PTSD". In WW I, the disorder was called "Shell Shock". In WWII and Korea, it was called "Combat Fatigue". Now it is called "Post Traumatic Stress Disorder", and mentally normal people today can't understand why some Vietnam Vets came home with it while others didn't. What is not understood about PTSD is that it happens to soldiers of all nations, even to those in the highly respected army of Israel. It also happens to non-military people, such as earthquake survivors, or civilians caught in wars.

As in bipolar disorder, the kindling process appears to be at work. Bipolar disorder and PTSD differ in stimulant, however. Bipolar disorder appears to develop from psychological blows having to do with loss of love, or threat of loss of love. PTSD, on the other hand, appears to develop from unspeakable threats of loss of life.[12] Here are a few examples of which I am personally aware:

- Adolescent boys in Vietnam enduring their first rocket attack and being forced to confront personal death before their brains are fully wired to deal with life's final chapter. For some, the terror is unendurable. They shot themselves, or fall on grenades.
- A Squad Leader sees two Vietnamese children, hand in hand, walking towards his squad. Around their necks are live hand grenades. The Squad Leader has Sophie's Choice: does he shoot the children, or does he let the children kill his squad? He shoots the children.
- A Medic's best friend asks to trade duty days. "No," says the Medic, "it's the most dangerous run. It's my turn." The friend insists. The Medic relents. The truck carrying the friend hits a mine. Despite the danger, the Medic rushes to his friend's assistance. No joy. The friend's head comes apart in the Medic's loving hands.

Such hideous inducing stimuli are repeated often during tours of duty in war, and they are suspected to play the role of Goddard's electricity in starting a kindling effect. a certain magnitude or number such stimulants are required to start the PTSD responses. Once started, the PTSD responses include hypervigilant fear, a greatly lowered auditory startle reaction, increased resting pulse rate and blood pressure, pronounced

---

12 Post, R.M. & Weiss, S.R.B. (1998), Sensitization and Kindling Phenomena in Mood, Anxiety, and Obsessive-Compulsive Disorders: The Role of Serotonergic Mechanisms in Illness Progression. *Biological Psychiatry, 44*: 193-206.

sleep disturbances, ceaseless ruminations of combat, recurrent flash-backs and nightmares[13] of unspeakable butcheries in both directions (that is, both as the receiver and as the butcher). Once the response begins, it becomes sensitive to non-war situations, such as close spaces, trails through forests, hunters shooting game, backfiring busses, or in the case of the Squad Leader cited above, any child of a certain age. While depression and panic attacks are common results of PTSD, mania is not. Nor are psychosis or illusions. Rather, the PTSD response seems to be one of involuntary mental transport back to past feelings of terrifying fear. Eventually, the response starts feeding upon itself. As in bipolar disorder, episodes beget episodes and the illness appears to become automatic.

In my bipolar disorder, I have experienced all the above mentioned PTSD responses even though I have never been in war. The final stimulus that kicked off my bipolar disorder was the threat of loss of my wife and family. I became so hypervigilantly fearful that the loss would occur that I could think of nothing else. Soon, a pronounced auditory startle reaction began. Telephone rings, the normal noise of an office at work, loud sounds on the TV, being unexpectedly spoken to by well-known co-workers made me startle. By the second year of my marriage crisis, my head pounded with headaches much of the time. I began measuring my blood pressure and pulse rate on drug store machines and discovered both to be well above my normal rates. Whenever I talked with my wife or my lawyer, my blood pressure and pulse rates shot up. I ceaselessly ruminated about my ex-wife's betrayal and my children's future until I began taking *valproic acid*, fourteen years after my illness began. Most interesting of all, my startle reaction is alive and well nineteen

---

13   No author cited, (1991),Teleconference. Neurobiological Alterations Associated With Post Traumatic Stress Disorder, National Center for PTSD, Clinical Laboratory and Education Division, Department of Veterans Affairs, White River Junction, VT., Palo Alto, Ca., Boston, Ma., West Haven, CT.

years after it began; in keeping with the predictions of the kindling effect and model, my startle reaction has become automatic. Even in sleep, even when listening to Bach, even in church, it erupts for no apparent reason.

The kindling phenomenon may also be at work in anxiety and fear. Pathological anxiety is the mother of anxiety disorders such as panic attacks, obsessive-compulsive disorder, and a range of phobias. While bipolar disorder is a mood illness, not an anxiety disorder, pathological anxiety nonetheless plays a major role in bipolar disorder. That is because the brain, in the course of constantly interacting with its environment, even in sleep, learns everything and forgets nothing. And because the part of the brain central to the circuits for fear, anxiety and pathological anxiety is (once again) the amygdala, known to be the regulator in short-term memory storage, the similarity in development of pathological anxiety and bipolar disorder appear strikingly similar.

Fear is, of course, normal and helpful. Fear responses, such as freezing in place, startling, pounding heart, soaring blood pressure and increased vigilance are appropriate defensives that can reduce danger by preparing a person either to engage the danger or to flee from it. Normal anxiety is also an appropriate defense to future "dangers", whether it be saving money for college or wanting to please a boss to remain secure in a job.

Pathological anxiety is, however, not normal. It is an exaggerated fear state that manifests itself in a highly negative affect associated with feelings that stability has been overwhelmed by uncertainty. Fear of being stalked by a raccoon is an example of pathological anxiety.

Rosen and Schulkin identify three general variables that may contribute to the development of hyperexcitability in the amygdala: genes, experience during critical stages in development, and physical or psychological trauma at any age. All three of those variables are components of the Post Model of bipolar disorder development. Using a partial kindling effect experiment (in which rat amygdalas were stimulated with tiny amounts of electricity), Rosen and Schulkin demonstrated that amygdalas might be stimulated into long lasting, even permanent states of hyperexcitability, short of seizures, that accelerate over time and eventually became autonomous. This experiment seems to indicate that the brain mechanisms responsible for hypervigilance of the environment, which stand to attention in a normal fear response, then return to normal once the fear is passed, perform differently once the pathological anxious state has been reached. In this hypothesis, repeated use of the synaptic connections in fear circuits causes the circuits to become efficient. Later they become permanent. Later still, they become automatic, that is, they become self-sustaining, no longer needing outside triggers to get them started.[14]

An example of this process in my experiences with bipolar disorder is a recurring anxiety dream that I have experienced all my life: *I open a door to a square room. Across the room is a second door that I must pass through. I have no choice. I absolutely must pass through it. In the exact center of the room, however, blocking my way with a sort of magical power, is a tiny piece of sponge dangling perfectly at lip-level from a string. I may not pass the sponge until it is eaten. At first, I am not troubled by the task. I simply put my lips around the sponge and pull it from the string (for some reason, I cannot use my hands). But when I eat the first piece of sponge, two more small sponges, dangling from strings as before, appear. By now, I am nauseous from the taste of the first sponge, and it bothers me that there are now two sponges where once there was one. But I have no choice. If I am to pass through the second door, which I must do, I must eat the two new sponges. I eat one of the two new ones with my lips, and two new sponges appear to replace it. The same happens for every piece of sponge that I eat, I eat by ones and the sponges reproduce by twos. I must*

---

14   Rosen, J.B. & Schulkin, Jay (1998). From Normal Fear to Pathological Anxiety. *Psychological Review, 105*, 2: 325-350.

eat them all, and soon the room is so full of tiny sponges that I can no longer breathe. I awaken, heart pounding, face sweating, gasping for air.

The dream is, of course, me nursing at my very anxious mother's breasts. It is an example of the synaptic connections in my fear circuits becoming efficient over time. Later they became permanent. Later still, they became automatic.

The Episodic Disorder

Post is not the only scientist whose work describes my illness. My symptoms are very similar to these described by neurologist Russell R. Monroe, which better describe my illness than does the DSM-IV in either the diagnosis of "Bipolar II" or "Brief Psychotic Disorder":

"The broadest generalization is that each [subject] experienced the precipitous onset of disturbed behavior with an equally abrupt remission that dramatically interrupted the life-style and life-flow of the individual. These "attacks" were recurrent and interspersed with long periods during which these individuals resumed their usual life-style.... The disturbed period could be as short as a few minutes to a few hours, but more often lasted for days, weeks or even several months, and commonly was associated with intense, unpleasant emotions characterized by fear, rage, depression, or a mixture of all of these and only rarely ecstatic feelings. Most commonly these episodic disorders included restlessness, agitation, sleeplessness, and racing thoughts, that is, disinhibited behavior; but on other occasions might have manifested inhibited behavior such as lethargy, apathy, difficulties in thinking or even muscular immobility and mutism. Other symptoms include confusion, illusions, hallucinations, and delusions, particularly paranoid delusions; bouts of neurotic symptoms such as panic or phobias; as well as physiologic changes, particularly rapid heart or regular heart beats, tremulousness, headaches, insomnia, weight changes, dizziness, and fainting spells."[15] (p. 207)

Monroe called his diagnosis, "Episodic Disorder." Later in his book, he identifies the illness that causes the disorder and locates the part of the brain in which it occurs:

"I have identified a specific biological marker, that is, focal epilepsy within the limbic system, as the most common correlate of this behavioral deviation." (p 228)

Then he adds:

Our current knowledge suggests that Vincent's [van Gogh] doctors were correct, he probably had seizural activity in the brain, that is, excessive firing of nerves; but this was focal and limited to the limbic system. If such firing had occurred in the area of the brain controlling motor functions, then Vincent would have experienced grand mal seizures. The fact that such abnormality was confined to the limbic system meant that Vincent did not have typical epilepsy, but, by intuition, his physicians were right in considering that he had epilepsy even without typical seizural symptoms." (p. 242)

I suspect that I suffer a similar illness not only because I recognize the symptoms of van Gogh's illness in myself, but also because I respond very well to the anti-convulsive drug (originally developed to contain epilepsy), *valproic acid*. As mentioned above, I was treated for fourteen years with *lithium carbonate* prior to going on *valproic acid* (in 1995). I did not respond to *lithium carbonate*; in fact, I almost committed suicide

---

15   Monroe, Russell R., *Creative Brainstorms*, ©1992, Irvington Publishers, Inc. New York City

in despair that I would ever be free of endless cycles of depression that continued despite my use of *lithium carbonate.*

Because of the stunning advances that Biological Psychiatry has made in understanding mental illness, it is tempting to declare that one science to be the Hero Science of mental illness. To do so, however, would be wholly wrong. The human brain/mind is far too complex to be understood by any single scientific discipline. For example, genetic inheritance clearly plays a role in certain mental illnesses. An afflicted person's environment is also a mighty determinant in mental illness, which crushes some people while others sail right through it. The genetic inheritances and the environmental experiences of *every* human are unique. It is clear therefore that *every* mind created by *every* brain is unique. Therefore, *every* eruption of mental illness is unique. Therefore, *every* individual's response to mental illness is unique. Therefore, *every* therapy (drugs and counseling) for mental illness must be unique.

For these reasons, among others, generalizations in mental health abound today as much as they did when neurologists were treating patients for "Masturbatory Insanity" and "Old Maid's Insanity". And it may very well be that no precise explanation will ever be developed. But though the Post Model is tentative, and though the Monroe diagnosis of "Episodic Disorder" has (to my knowledge) never been tested (with the implantation of electrodes in the limbic system of someone like me), I prefer both to my psychiatric diagnosis of "Bipolar II Disorder". That is because Neurology and Biological Psychiatry are hard sciences is "hard science" while clinical psychiatry (meaning the implied "science" greater than medical doctor training) and all its various psychologies are "soft sciences". By this I mean that Neurology and Biological Psychiatry attempts to define my illness by direct measurement of *neuron (brain cell) behavior,* while clinical psychiatry and its plethora of psychologies attempt to categorize and treat my illness by observed (read, "subjective") *personality behavior.*

The Continuum of Mental Illness

Carl Menninger conceived of mental illness as a continuum of social incompatibility, a concept that resonates strongly with my experiences. Schizophrenics, for example, are almost totally withdrawn from society. Psychotics mostly are. The moods disturbed and depressed sometimes are. Those with behavior problems do not withdraw but participate poorly.

If there is a continuum of social incompatibility is there also a continuum of illnesses—are schizophrenia, psychosis, acute mania, bipolar and unipolar depression, epilepsy behavioral syndrome and epilepsy all different manifestations of the same illness? Evidence from research appears to confirm this possibility. Suspected genes for schizophrenia and bipolar disorder have been found to overlap.[16] Structural studies of the brains of schizophrenics and bipolars have been found "more affected in schizophrenia" and "subtle" in mood disorders.[17] Some drugs work very well for schizophrenia and acute mania.[18] Electrical kindling (of epilepsy) is most readily achieved in limbic system structures, the same structures that are thought to be important in affective disorders.[19] Drugs that work well for epilepsy work very well for mood disorders.[20] Finally, depression and mania are, of course, closely twined in bipolar disorder.

---

16   Berrettini, W.H., 2000, Susceptibility loci for bipolar disorder: overlap with inherited vulnerability to schizophrenia. *Biological Psychiatry*, February 1; 47(3): 245-51

17   Baumann, B. & Bogerts, B., 1999. The pathomorphology of schizophrenia and mood disorders: similarities and differences. *Schizophr Res* Sep 29; 39(2): 141-8

18   Post, R.M., 1999. Comparative pharmacology of bipolar disorder and schizophrenia. *Schizophr Res Sep 29*; 39(2):153-8; discussion 163

19   Weiss, S.R. & Post, R.M. 1998. Kindling: spearate vs. shared mechanisms in affective disorders and epilepsy. *Neuropsychobiology*, Oct; 38(3): 167-80

20   Post, R.M.; Ketter, T.A.; Denicoff, P.J; Pazzaglia, P.J.; Leverich, G.S.; Marangell, L.B.; Callahan, A.M.; George, M.S.; Frye, M.A., (1996). The place of anticonvulsant therapy in bipolar illness. *Psychopharmacology 128*: 115-129.

But, as has been observed elsewhere in this book, nothing is simple about the human brain. Affective disorders secondary to neurological disorders also erupt. These neurological disorders include Traumatic Brain Injury, which often yields depression and/or mania. Stroke and depression are common. Wilson's Disease is sometimes complicated with anxiety, mood disorders and psychosis. Brain Tumors and depression have been linked. Multiple Sclerosis, depression, mania, and a high rate of suicide have been reported. Parkinson's and Huntington's Diseases often present with depression, anxiety, panic attacks and hallucinations.[21] Because each of these neurological disorders involves a different part of the brain, the moods and psychoses they excite might form a map of where in the brain nascent moods and psychoses reside. If the various illnesses do indeed reside in different parts of the brain, can mental illnesses be considered a continuum of the same illness? I have found no answer to this question in my research. My personal suspicion is that the mental illnesses will be found to connect, just as every in the brain connects, but not as a continuum. It seems to me that my mental illness began as an illness of memory, then graduated into involuntary brain spasms not unlike involuntary muscle spasms.

---

21   Gauze, B.H. & Gitlin, M. (1994). The neuropathologic basis of major affective disorders: neuroanatomic insights. *Journal of Neuropsychiatry 6 (2)*: 114-121

2

Genetics

History

Genetics is "the science of variation and heredity"; where heredity is not the money and property inherited from dead relatives, but their biology, such as noses, teeth and hair.[22] This science began in 1866 (just five years after Wilhelm Griesinger first saw the nerves and cells of the nervous system through a microscope) with the observations of Gregor Mendel, an Austrian priest. From careful observations of flowering garden peas, Mendel postulated that pairs of hereditary factors account for all development in organisms that reproduce sexually. He was right, of course. What he called "hereditary factors" we now call "genes". His discovery, however, described a very simple organism and a very simple experiment—crossing red-flowered peas with white-flowered peas.

Although the stirrings of modern genetics began with Mendel, the science took form in the 1930's, when a medical doctor from Russia, named Aaron Rosanoff, undertook the first large-scale twin study using data from the California State Hospitals.

There are, of course, identical twins and fraternal twins. Identical twins have exactly the same genetic inheritance, while fraternal twins are no more alike than brothers and sisters. Theoretically, therefore, a

---

22   Barnett, S. A., 1998. *The Science of Life.* Allen & Unwin, St. Leonards 2065 Australia.

genetic cause of serious mental illness could be proven if both members of an identical twin set developed an illness, and disproved if only one did. Conversely, if both twins in a fraternal set developed a serious mental illness, a genetic cause could be disproved.

Rosanoff identified 1,014 pairs of twins in which one twin had a major mental illness. Schizophrenia was diagnosed in 142 of the pairs. Among the identical twins, both twins developed schizophrenia in 68.3 percent of the cases. Among the fraternal twins, both twins developed schizophrenia in only 14.9 percent of the cases.

Rosanoff also looked at 90 twin pairs who developed manic-depressive illness. For identical twins, the second twin also got ill in 69.6 percent of the cases. For fraternal twin pairs, the second twin also got ill in 16.4 percent of the cases.[23]

In science, others must duplicate all results before they are fully accepted. Rosanoff's results were duplicated in 1945, when Franz Kallmann studied 73,000 patients of the public asylums in the state of New York. Kallmann identified 691 schizophrenics with a traceable co-twin. For the identical twins, the second twin was also ill in 85.8 percent of the cases. For the fraternal twins, the second twin was also ill in only 14.7 percent of the cases.[24]

Next came the Danish adoption study of Seymour Kety, which took a different tack from the twin studies of Rosanoff and Kallmann.

The state of Denmark follows its citizens precisely through life. An adoption register of the State Department of Justice permits researchers to identify the biological relatives of children who are adopted. A population register makes it possible to locate the children who are adopted and to follow their life histories. In Denmark, therefore, one is able to study the biological background of adopted children as well as their subsequent medical fates.

---

23   Shorter, E., (1997). *A History of Psychiatry*, New York, NY: John Wiley & Sons, Inc., p242
24   *ibid*, p243

In 1968, Kety and collaborators published the results of their Denmark study of 5,483 adoptions in Copenhagen between 1924 and 1947. From this group, 507 adopted children were later admitted to a psychiatric hospital. Independent observers reviewed their case histories [note the subjectivity] and identified 33 of them as schizophrenics. These patients and their biological families were then compared with an age-matched control group of adopted children and their biological families who had never been admitted to a psychiatric hospital. Within the biological families of the adopted schizophrenics, the illness was found to exist in about 10 percent of their closest biological relatives. Within the biological families of the adopted children never admitted to a psychiatric hospital, there was very little schizophrenia. This study appears to show that schizophrenia is somewhat genetic. Note, however, that environmental factors in the schizophrenics were not studied.[25]

Modern Genetics

Now, 134 years after Gregor Mendel postulated "pairs of hereditary factors" at work in his garden peas, a rough, generic draft of the total genetic constitution of the human species, its genome, has been completed.[26] In your mind, stress "generic", for each of us are variations on the basic sequence of the genome, and therein lies our tales, for a single gene can be responsible for a great complexity of functions. For example, it is the function of genes to encode the structure of proteins that do the work of life and a single gene can encode or modify perhaps 10 or more protein structures, each varying in the amount and combination of instructions that they in turn give a cell. Also, genes are known to act in multiples. There is not likely to be a single gene discovered to account for any mental illness, nor for intelligence, nor for moral

---

25   ibid, p244
26   Baltimore, D., "50,000 Genes and We Know Them All (Almost)" *New York Times,* 25 June 2000, Op-Ed Page.

worth, nor for special skills.[27] Furthermore, genes react to environ-
ments. Depending upon the soil in which they grow, genetically identical oak trees might develop into scrub oaks or mighty giants. Likewise,
the same person who fails as an inner-city street urchin might flourish
in the more stable environment of an Iowa farm community.[28] Finally,
genes mutate, not least because of the constant bombardment of cos-
mic rays that pass through us every moment. Therefore, a person's
genes may not be the same from one hour to the next.

Given its Medusa-like complexity, then, what may be said about
modern genetics and the light of understanding that it sheds upon
mental illness?

First, progress is being made. The following annotations from recent
genetic research literature shows a science making steady and cautious
progress:

> **1989:** Bipolar affective disorder appears to be a heterogeneous
> ["mixed"] disorder with multiple independently inherited
> disease genes, each giving similar clinical results (bipolar,
> unipolar, and other disorders).[29]

> **1991:** The results overall suggest that a gene predisposing to
> manic-depression (bipolar affective illness) localized on the
> X-chromosome may exists in a subgroup of bipolar cases.[30]

> **1993:** Many of the recent studies reporting genetic linkages
> for mental illnesses such as schizophrenia and manic-depres-
> sion have been retracted.[31]

---

27 Barnett, S. A., 1998. *The Science of Life.* Allen & Unwin, St. Leonards 2065
    Australia.1998,
28 *ibid*, p64
29 Gershon, E.S., (1989). Recent developments in genetics of manic-depressive ill-
    ness. *Journal of Clinical Psychiatry 50, [12 Suppl]*: 4-7.
30 Baron, M., (1991). X-linkage and manic-depressive illness: a reassessment. *Soc.-
    Biol. 38, 3-4*: 179-188.
31 Alper, J.S. & Natowicz, M.R., (1993). On establishing the genetic basis of mental
    disease. *Trends-Neuroscience: 16, 19*: 387-389.

1994: On the whole, linkage and association studies contributed to the localization of some potential vulnerability genes for manic-depression on chromosome X and 11, and more recently, 18.[32]

1997: The authors present a review of published studies which suggest that it is presently unclear whether one or more susceptibility loci on chromosome 18 exist, and that their more accurate localization is unknown.[33]

1997: Efforts to understand the mechanisms of inheritance have been hindered by the complexity of the phenotype [a polite way of saying that it's hard to be objective about subjective diagnoses], which may range from benign mood swings to chronic psychosis, and by apparently non-Mendelian modes of transmission.[34]

1998: Advances in the human genetic map and in genetic analysis of linkage and association in complex inheritance traits have led to genetic progress in these major psychoses. For chromosome 6 in schizophrenia and for chromosomes 18 and 21 in manic-depressive illness, there are reports of linkage in several independent data sets...but convincing associations remain to be demonstrated.[35]

---

32 Souery, D.; Mendelbaum, K. & Mendlewicz, J. (1994). Genetics and manic-depressive psychosis: review and current findings. *Acta Psychiatr Belg. 94, 3*: 134-150.

33 Ewald, H.: Mors, O.; Koed, K.; Eiberg, H.; Kruse, T.A., (1997). Susceptibility loci for bipolar affective disorder on chromosome 18? A review and study of Danish families. *Psychiatric-Genetics 7, 1*: 1-12.

34 MacKinnon, D.F.; Jamison, Kay Redfield; DePaulo, J.R., (1997). Genetics of manic depressive illness. *Annual Review of Neuroscience 20*: 355-373.

35 Gershon, E.S.; Badner, J.A.; Goldin, L.R.; Sanders, A.R.; Cravchik, A.; Detera, W.; Sevilla, D., (1998). Closing in on genes for manic-depressive illness and schizophrenia. *Neuropsychopharmacology 18, 4*: 233-242.

1999: Previous reported linkage of bipolar affective disorder to DNA markers on chromosome 18 was reexamined in a large sample of German bipolar families...Evidence for linkage was obtained for chromosomal region 18p11.2 in the paternal families and for 18q22-23 in the 'either' families. The findings on 18p11.2 and 18q22-23 support prior evidence for susceptibility loci in these regions.[36]

2000: Recent genetic linkage studies have defined confirmed susceptibility loci for bipolar disorder for multiple regions of the human genome, including 4p16, 12q24, 18p11.2, 18q22, 21q21, 22q11-13, and Xq26. Studies of schizophrenia kindred have yielded robust evidence for susceptibility at 18p11.2 and 22q11-13, both of which are implicate in susceptibility to bipolar disorder. Similarly, confirmed schizophrenia vulnerability loci have been mapped for 6p24, 8p and 13q32. Strong statistical evidence for a 13q32 bipolar disorder susceptibility locus has been reported. Thus, both family and molecular studies of these disorders suggest shared genetic susceptibility. These two groups of disorders may not be so distinct as current [classification] suggests.[37]

Secondly, the astounding progress in understanding genetics has encouraged insupportable simplification. *Nothing* about genes is simple. Each gene is like an individual history book of life on earth. Just as it is impossible to say, "This is a history book" and communicate the

---

36   Nothen, M.M.; Chchon, S. Rohleder, H.; Hemmer, S.; Franzek, E.; Fritze, J.; Albus, M.; Borrmann-Hassenbach, M.; Kreiner, R.; Weigelt, B.; Minges, J.; Lichermann, D.; Maier, W.; Craddock, N.; Frimmers, R.; Holler, T.; Baur, M.P.; Rietchel, M.; Propping, P. (1999). *Molecular Psychiatry, 4 (1)*: 76-84.

37   Berrettini, W.H., 2000. Susceptibility loci for bipolar disorder: overlap with inherited vulnerability to schizophrenia. *Biological Psychiatry*, February 1; 47(3): 245-51

book's contents, so it is with saying, "This is a gene". If we were to look backward into the history of individual genes, we would start with meiosis, the awe-inspiring process by which, say, 50,000 genes from the mother are mixed with another 50,000 genes from the father. Some of the resulting sum of 100,000 genes is selected in for the new human, and some is selected out. This is where the finger of God touches us. This is where we become ourselves, for when the process is complete, each of us (except for identical twins) has a unique set of 50,000 random genes, an inheritance that reaches back in history to the first life forms that populated the earth. It does so because that is what happens in a closed system such as the earth. Everything is recycled forever, even the DNA of the Blue-Green Algae, the life form that "discovered" sexual reproduction. Without doubt, particles of my DNA once existed in a caveman, and in Scots and Englishmen, some of whom might have fought with Henry V "Upon St. Crispin's Day". Yet, those of my brother may have totally different histories. As it is in this history metaphor, so it is in function—each person's unique collection of genes will function uniquely. I have developed mental illness and my brother has developed ulcers. *Nothing* about genes is simple.

3

Clinical Psychiatry

History

The concept of "psychiatry" arose in the asylum era, not with the first asylum-keepers that kept their charges in chains, but with the asylum-keepers of the Enlightenment Period that developed the idea that humane confinement in asylums could be therapy for mental illness. In London, the Priory of St. Mary of Bethlehem (a name corrupted first into "Bethlem", then into "Bedlam") housed the insane at least as early as 1403. In 1656, Louis XIV created the *Salpetriere* and *Becetre* hospices for "the sick, the criminal, the homeless and the insane". The rest of Europe favored the "madhouse" concept, which resembled joint ventures between the state, church and local communities.

The idea of "asylum as therapy" began with an English "Mad-Doctor", William Battie, who published in 1758 a *Treatise on Madness*, in which he attributed therapeutic virtues to the asylum concept. "Madness," he wrote, "is...as manageable as many other distempers, which are equally dreadful and obstinate, and yet are not looked upon as incurable; such unhappy objects ought by no means to be abandoned, much less shut up in loathsome prisons as criminals or nuisances to the society."[38]

---

38   Shorter, E., (1997). *A History of Psychiatry*, New York, NY: John Wiley & Sons, Inc., p10

The idea grew. In 1788, in Florence, Italy, Vicenzio Chiarugi opened the Bonifazio mental hospital. This is the first such asylum where the staff was given written instructions for dealing with their inmates in a humane way. This may also have been the first asylum in which the inmates were unchained.

The founder of "Psychiatry", however, is considered to be Philippe Pinel, who gained his experience at the *Bicetre* and *Salpetriere*. In a text-book that he published in 1801, Pinel wrote, "The hope is well-justified of returning to society individuals who seem to be hopeless. Our most assiduous and unflagging attention is required toward that numerous group of psychiatric patients who are convalescening or are lucid between episodes, a group that must be placed in the separate ward of the hospice...and subjected to a kind of psychological treatment for the purpose of developing and strengthening their faculties of reason."[39]

Then came, in 1861, the first step of the modern biopsychiatric revolution. Through a microscope, Griesinger saw the nerves and cells of the brain. The hard wiring of the brain was revealed. Brain science was underway.

The path to the biopsychiatric revolution was, however, lumpy. Soon after Griesinger, two more German neurologists whipsawed psychiatry between them. Emil Kraepelin, an asylum-keeper, conceptualized the major classifications of mental illness in 1893, and Sigmund Freud began introducing his mind-science, "Psychoanalysis", with the publication of his book on dreams in 1900. Psychiatry first embraced the conceptual breakthroughs of Kraepelin, which related to the serious mental illnesses, then rushed pell-mell to embrace the neurosis ideas of Freud, which related to the less serious mental illnesses, such as hysteria and situational depression. The asylum methods of Pinel and Kraepelin were not totally abandoned when Freudianism took over psychiatry.

---

39   *Ibid*, p 12

Asylums were still used for the most seriously ill–the schizophrenics and the manic-depressives. But for everyone else with "personality disorders" there was the Freudian Couch and the fifty-minute hour.

I find it easy to be critical of Freud and of the psychiatrists who rushed to embrace his methods. First of all, Freud openly admitted that his methods would do nothing for psychotics (schizophrenics and manic-depressives). They were hopeless as far as he was concerned. His "science" was for the understanding and cure of neuroses, also called personality disorders. Secondly, Freud's division of the human mind into "Id, Ego and Superego" is astoundingly similar to Plato's. In his *Republic,* Plato philosophized about two warring elements in humans that he called "desire" and "reason". What, Plato pondered, kept desire from dominating reason? Plato hypothesized a third element, which he called the *thymos,* which he conceived as the executive arm of reason to enforce its decisions. Substitute "Id" for desire, "Ego" for reason and "Superego" for *thymos* and you might, like me, suspect that Freud failed to cite Plato. Thirdly, Freud's organizing idea, that we spend our adulthoods working out the problems of our childhoods, was said first by the English poet, William Wordsworth in 1807–"The child is the father of the man". Fourthly, Freudian methods are premised on the idea that a superior mind guides a troubled mind to "normalcy". Now that real science has revealed what the mind really is, it seems humorous to me that anyone can claim to have a "superior" one. Fifthly, who wouldn't prefer to work in a private office than an asylum?

However, neurotic people are entitled to all the attention they care to pay for. And had I been a psychiatrist in 1900, I would have been swept up in the "new method". It would have seemed a very humane way to treat the personality disordered. Therefore, I will judge Freud by his time, not by my own.

Psychoanalysis crested in the USA in the 1960's then began to decline. In general, it is, today, just another psychology therapy in a quiver of 250 or so others. Given the brave new worlds of genetics and psychopharmacology, it can't be anything more; but like an old sin, it continues to cast a long shadow. One of these days, when a psychiatrists tells me that my depression is "anger turned inward", I am going scream, throw a tantrum, then suddenly stop and say, "Ah! See how my unresolved childhood sexual conflicts disrupt my adulthood".

For all my negative feeling about Freud, I do not take him lightly. Some of his insights have been very helpful to me in rebuilding my smashed "mind". In my experience, however, while his insights pointed towards an understanding of my disordered mind, they did not provide containment of the recurring depression that almost killed me.

One incontrovertible thing that can be said for Freud is that his methods created the medical specialty called "clinical psychiatry", which is, because it diagnoses mental illnesses and prescribes drugs accordingly, essential to the mentally ill.

Clinical psychiatrists attain their position by attending medical school for four years. Then, as a M.D. (doctor of medicine), they receive additional training during a psychiatric residency of three or four years. In a sense, clinical psychiatrists use their medical training when applying the drugs that biopsychiatry discovers and their psychiatric residency training in diagnosis of the mentally ill and in applying the plethora of counseling therapies available. As a profession, they have carried forward Kraepelin's concept of classifications in their Bible of mental illness diagnoses called *Diagnostic and Statistical Manual,* abbreviated "DSM". The DSM has gone through four editions, which are called, respectfully, "DSM-I, DSM-II, DSM-III, and DSM-IV".

The DSM series grew out of a publication called *Statistical Manual for the Use of Institutions for the Insane,* which was issued in 1918 by the American Medico-Psychological Association. Until 1952, that was the only Kraepelin-like diagnostic tool available in the United States. In1952, however, the American Psychiatric published its DSM-I and America had a new diagnostic standard. The DSM-I listed 106 diagnoses. By 1960 the Freudians, who dominated American psychiatry, were unhappy with DSM-I. They lead the committee that published, in 1968, the DSM-II. Much more strongly Freudian, the DSM-II listed 180 diagnoses. But by the time the DSM-II was published, the Freudians were rowing against the tide of biopsychiatry. Very effective drugs for schizophrenia, anxiety, depression and mania were already on the market and more were in the pipeline. The great Freudian wave had crested and was being sucked into the next one, that of biopsychiatry. Obviously another DSM was needed, something completely different, something that would reposition psychiatry out of the Freud camp and into that of biopsychiatry.

Published in 1980, the DSM-III did succeed in beginning, but not completing, the turning away of the series from Freud's model into biopsychiatry. The diagnostician's "best clinical judgement and experience", was replaced with standardized diagnoses that would theoretically not vary in use regardless of practitioner and result in accurate drug and counseling therapies. But while standardization was aimed at, no one knows if it was achieved. No blind study of clinical psychiatrists diagnosing the same mentally ill persons was ever done.

There were other problems. Critics called it ethnocentric, claiming that "anorexia nervosa" was a diagnosis found only in the U.S.A. Others complained that it was still Freudian because it retained Freudian terms such as "neurosis". Others pointed to "political diagnoses", such as the homosexuality diagnosis once called "sexual deviation" that disappeared in 1974. Others pointed to the sudden appearance, in 1978, following the Vietnam War, of "Post Traumatic Stress Syndrome". How, they asked, could politics determine science?

To answer criticism such as this, the APA plunged once more into the breech and published, in 1994, the DSM-IV. Diagnosis creep continued. DSM-I had 106 diagnoses. DSM-II had 180 diagnoses. DSM-III had 265 diagnoses. DSM-IV has 297 diagnoses. That's a 180 % increase in diagnoses in 16 years, an average increase of 12 new diagnoses per year.

Can any clinical psychiatrist master 297 separate diagnoses even with the help of a Bible?

Finally, however, the ghost of Freud was exorcised. In the DSM-IV, there are no diagnoses with "neurosis" in their names. Gone, too, was Kraepelin's classification of "Manic-Depression" as a psychosis, replaced with the term "Bipolar disorder" and classified under "Mood Disorders". Kraepelin's single diagnosis of *praecox dementia* has been exploded into five different kinds of schizophrenia and seven other types of psychotic illnesses. There are six Bipolar I diagnoses and three Bipolar II diagnoses. There are eleven Anxiety Diagnoses. Seven Somatoform Diagnoses. Two Facitious Diagnoses. Five Dissociative Diagnoses. Twenty-nine Sexual and Gender Identity Diagnoses. Three Eating Diagnoses. Thirteen Primary Sleep Diagnoses. Six Impulse-Control Diagnoses Not Elsewhere Classified. Six Adjustment Diagnoses. Eleven Personality Diagnoses, and thirty-two "Other Conditions That May Be a Focus of Clinical Attention".

I have many reservations about the book that has been used to classify me. First and most importantly, no blind study has ever been done to test the validity of the diagnoses. Granted, MRI's can't see mental illness. Judgement is still required. But if a medical specialty publishes a book represented to assist in medical judgement, shouldn't there be a scientific attempt to validate whether it succeeded?

Secondly, in my research I have come across two diagnostic instruments that, in my opinion, represent better diagnostic science than that found in the DSM-IV. The first is a decision tree called, "Schedule for Affective Disorders and Schizophrenia, Life-time Version".[40] The second is the National Institute of Mental Health Life Chart Methodology.[41]

---

40   Spitzer, R.L., Endicott, J., (1979) *Schedule for Affective Disorders and Schizophrenia-Life-time Version*, Research Assessment and Training Unit, New York State Psychiatric Institute, NYC.

41   Leverich, G.S. & Post, R.M., (1998). Life charting of affective disorders. *The International Journal of Neuropsychiatric Medicine, 3* (5): 21-37

Both of these instruments are strongly Kraepelin in that they systematically structure a patient's symptoms into a visual representation of their illness, from which scientific management becomes possible.

Finally, add me to the category of the little boy who observed that the Emperor had no clothes: I just plain don't believe that there are 297 mental and behavioral disorders. A far more common sense system of categorization, in my opinion, is that created by the neurologist Russell R. Monroe.[42]

Russell Monroe's Classification System

1. The Major Psychoses

A. Schizophrenia

B. Bipolar Disease

2. The Mild Psychoses

A. Episodic Disorders: The disturbed period can be as short as a few minutes to a few hours, but more often lasts for a day, a week or even for several months. It is commonly associated with intense, unpleasant emotions characterized by fear, rage, depression, or a mixture of all of these and only rarely ecstatic feelings. Most commonly these episodic disorders included restlessness, agitation, sleeplessness, and racing thoughts, that is, disinhibited behavior; but on other occasions they might manifest inhibited behavior such as lethargy, apathy, difficulties in thinking or even muscular immobility and mutism. Other symptoms include confusion, illusions, hallucinations, and delusions, particularly paranoid delusions; bouts of neurotic symptoms such as panic or phobias; as well as physiologic changes, particularly rapid heart or irregular heart beats,

---

42   Monroe, Russell R., *Creative Brainstorms*, ©1992, Irvington Publishers, Inc. New York, New York

tremulousness, headaches, insomnia, weight changes, dizziness, and fainting spells. (p. 207)

B. Paranoid Disorders: Chronic mental disorders in which there has been an insidious development of a permanent and unshakeable delusional system (persecutory delusions or delusions of jealousy), accompanied by preservation of clear and orderly thinking. Emotional responses and behavior are consistent with the delusional state.[43]

3. Borderline Syndrome

A. Pan Anxiety: The unpleasant emotional state consisting of psychophysiological responses to anticipation of unreal or imagined danger, ostensibly resulting from unrecognized intrapsychic conflict. Physiological concomitants include increased heart rate, altered respiration rate, sweating, trembling, weakness and fatigue, psychological concomitants include feelings of impending danger, powerlessness, apprehension and tension.[44]

B. Pan Neurosis: a mental and emotional disorder that affects only part of the personality, is accompanied by a less distorted perception of reality than in a psychosis, does not result in disturbance of the use of language, and is accompanied by various physical, physiological, and mental disturbances (as visceral symptoms, anxieties, or phobias).[45]

C. Depersonalization: An alteration in the perception of the self so that the usual sense of one's own reality is lost, manifested in a sense of unreality or self-estrangement, in changes

---

43   © *On-line Medical Dictionary*

44   *Ibid*

45   WWWebster Dictionary copyright © 2000 by Merriam-Webster, Incorporated

of body image, or in a feeling that one does not control his own actions and speech.[46]

D. Plus: a transient overt psychotic (detachment from reality) episode

E. Plus: loneliness, emptiness, and hopelessness

4. The Neuroses

A. Loss of Ego Boundaries: "Disintegration of Self".

B. Estrangement from the world

C. De-realization: Living in dream-like states.

D. Depersonalization: Loss of self-identity.

5. The Behavior Disorders

No doubt about it, Monroe's system is partially Freudian, but that is just fine. There are many Freudian concepts that are still accurate in the biopsychiatric era. What appeals to me most in Monroe's system is that it matches the fruits of biopsychiatry better than the DSM-IV. Assuming that it is generally true that behavior disorders can't be cured or contained with drugs, Monroe's diagnoses exactly match the common drugs developed by biopsychiatry, which are, according to Microsoft's *Encarta Encyclopedia:*

Category	*Drug Class*	*Generic Name*	*Trade Name*
Antipsychotic drugs	Phenothiazines	chlorpromazine	Thorazine
		fluphenazine	Prolixin
		thioridazine	Mellaril
		trifluoperazine	Stelazine
	Thioxanthenes	chlorprothixene	Taractin

---

46   © *On-line Medical Dictionary*

		thiothixene	Navane
	Benzisoxazole derivatives	risoridone	Risperdal
	Butryophenones	haloperidon	Haldol
	Dibenzodiazephines	clozapine	Clozaril
	Dibenzoxazepines	loxapine	Loxitane
	Dihydroindolines	molindone	Moban
	Thienobenzodia-zephines	olanzapine	Zyprexa
Antimanic drugs	Lithium salts	lithium carbonate	Eskalith
	Iminostibenes	carbamazepine	Tegretol
	Carbolic acids	valproate	Depakene
Antidepressant drugs	Tricyclics	amitriptyline	Elavil
		clomipramine	Anafranil
		desipramine	Norpramin
		doxepin	Sinequan
		impramine	Tofranil
		nortriptyline	Pamelor
		protriptyline	Vivactil
	Tetracyclics	maprotiline	Ludiomil
	Selective serotonin reuptake inhibitors	fluoxetine	Prozac
		paroxetine	Paxil
		sertraline	Zoloft

	Dopamine reuptake inhibitors	bupropion	Wellbutrin
	Monoamine oxidase (MAO) inhibitors	phenelzine	Nardil
Antianxiety drugs	Benzodiazepines	alprazolam	Xanax
		chlordiazepoxide	Librium
		clonazepam	Klonopin
		clorazepate	Tranxene
		diazepam	Valium
		halazepam	Paxipam
		lorazepam	Ativan
		oxazepam	Serax
	Azaspiro-decanediones	buspirone	BuSpar
	Propanediol carbamates	meprobamate	Miltown

Furthermore, Monroe's diagnosis of "Episodic Disorder", as noted earlier, far better describes my illness than do the one called "Bipolar II Mood Disorder" and "Brief Psychotic Disorder". Here is a comparison between diagnostic criteria found in Monroe's "Episodic Disorder" and that called "Bipolar II" in the DSM-IV. I have marked in **bold** those descriptions of Monroe's not found in the DSM-IV.

Monroe's Episodic Disorder:

- "It is commonly associated with intense, unpleasant emotions characterized by **fear, rage**, depression, or a mixture of all of these and only **rarely ecstatic feelings.**"
- "[it includes] **restlessness, agitation, sleeplessness,** and **racing thoughts…**"

- "But on other occasions, they might manifest inhibited behavior such as **lethargy, apathy, difficulties in thinking** or even **muscular immobility…**"
- "Other symptoms include **confusion…dizziness…**"

The DSM-IV's Bipolar II diagnosis:
- The essential feature of Bipolar II Disorder is a clinical course that is characterized by the occurrence of one or more Major Depressive Episodes (Criterion A) accompanied by at least one Hypomanic Episode (Criterion B).
- Hypomanic Episodes should not be confused with the several days of euthymia that may follow remission of a Major Depressive Episode. The presence of a Manic or Mixed Episode precludes the diagnosis of Bipolar II Disorder (Criterion C).
- Episodes of Substance-Induced Mood Disorder (due to the direct psysiological effects of a medication, other somatic treatments for depression, drugs of abuse, or toxin exposure) or of Mood Disorder Due to a General Medical Condition do not count toward a diagnosis of Bipolar II Disorder.
- In addition, the episodes must not be better accounted for by Schizoaffective Disorder and are not superimposed on Schizophrenia, Schizophreniform Disorder, Delusional Disorder, or Psychotic Disorder Not Otherwise Specified (Criterion D).
- The symptoms must cause clinically significant distress or impairment in social, occupational, or other important areas of functioning (Criterion E).
- In come cases, the Hypomanic Episodes themselves do not cause impairment. Instead, the impairment may result from the Major Depressive Episodes or from a chronic pattern of unpredictable mood episodes and fluctuating unreliable interpersonal or occupational functioning.

- Individuals with Bipolar II Disorder may not view the Hypomanic Episodes as pathological, although others may be troubled by the individuals' erratic behavior. Often individuals, particularly when in the midst of a Major Depressive Episode, do not recall periods of hypomania without reminders from close friends or relatives. Information from other informants is often critical in establishing the diagnosis of Bipolar II Disorder.[47]

I agree that I meet all of the criteria for the DSM-IV diagnosis, "Bipolar II". But Russell Monroe's Episodic Disorder describes my experiences far more accurately.

How then to summarize clinical psychiatry's place in the biopsychiatric era? One critic has called it "a science attempting to define itself"[48] I am tempted to subscribe to that idea. How can a "scientific discipline" be a discipline when each of its practitioners has 297 separate diagnoses, thirty-eight common drugs, a minimum of four major psychotherapies to master and a medical economy that forces them to see many patients in a short amount of time?

Yet, the medical training of the profession is definitely scientific and, at the entirely practical level, they control the drugs that someone like me must have. Therefore, whether or not clinical psychiatry is a science it is indispensable in the biopsychiatric era.

A final word on the history of the profession. It is clear, today, that the lasting revolutionary of the time when clinical psychiatry gave birth to itself was Kraepelin, not Freud. Prior to Kraepelin, mental illness diagnoses included such nonsense as "masturbatory insanity", "wedding-night psychosis", "chronic delusional disorder", "old maid's insanity", "moon madness", "monomania", and the like. Using color-coded

---

47 *Diagnostic and Statistical Manual of Mental Disorders, Forth Edition, p 359.* (1994). Washington DC, American Psychiatric Association.

48 Shorter, E., (1997). *A History of Psychiatry*, New York, NY: John Wiley & Sons, Inc.

cards and a computer-like mind, Kraepelin and his staff charted the severity and characteristics of each patient's episodes. Then he deduced from his copious data two major mental illnesses. The first he named *dementia praecox* (later "Schizophrenia"). The second he named "Manic Depression". As a testament to how completely he described manic-depression, no new characteristic of the illness has been added since he first described it. The characteristics that he deduced include euphoric and dysphoric (sad) mania, melancholic and agitated depression, manic and depressive stupor, and the tremendous variability in the evolution of the illness including rapid and ultrarapid cycling. At least in the realm of mental illness science, Kraepelin's leaps of insight may be equated to those of Newton and Watson and Crick. That is because today, 104 years later, the sciences of mental illness are following the path that the Good Dr. Kraepelin set for it in 1893.

Not bad for a near-sighted guy who couldn't use a microscope.

Diagnosis

The first formidable hurdle that a psychiatrist faces in treating the mentally ill is diagnosis, which is always a subjective judgement based upon the cultural and personal behavior of the patient observed through the filters of the cultural and personal biases of the psychiatrist. There are no CAT Scans, DNA or blood tests that can pinpoint what is going on in the brain/mind of a human. Rather, the psychiatrist must make a diagnosis based upon his or her knowledge of biology and the social, economic and cultural conditions in which the patient lives. The DSM-IV lists thirteen classifications of mental and behavioral disorders and 297 separate disorders. Because these numbers are so great, it is easiest for patients like me to consider the disorders by category.

Without question, the most debilitating category of mental disorder is "Schizophrenia and Psychoses". These disorders cause lost contact with reality. Symptoms may include delusions and hallucinations, disorganized thinking and speech, bizarre behavior, a diminished range of emotions and social withdrawal.

"Mood Disorders" (also called "Affective Disorders") is a category of major illnesses that disrupt a person's emotional life. Depression, mania, unipolar and bipolar disorders are examples of mood disorders.

The Anxiety Disorders begin the less-major illnesses. These disorders include panic attacks, agoraphobia and phobias.

"Somatoform Disorders" are characterized by the presence of physical symptoms that cannot be explained by a medical condition or another mental illness. Thus, psychiatrists often judge that such symptoms result from psychological conflicts or distress. For example, in conversion disorder, once called "hysteria", a person may experience blindness, deafness, or seizures, but a psychiatrist cannot find anything wrong with the person.[49]

The "Factitious Disorders" category contains illnesses characterized by physical or psychological symptoms that are not real, genuine, or natural.[50]

The Dissociative Disorders are sudden temporary alterations in the normally integrative functions of consciousness.[51]

The Sexual and Gender Identity Disorders include, but are not limited to, Hypoactive Sexual Desire, Sexual Aversion, Exibitionism, Sadism, Transvestic Fetishism, etc.

The Eating Disorders category contains the behavioral disorders, Anorexia Nervosa and Bulimia Nervosa.

The Sleep Disorders include, but are not limited to, Insomnia, Hypersomnia, Narcolepsy, Sleep Terror, Sleepwalking, etc.

---

49   "Mental Illness," *Microsoft® Encarta® Encyclopedia 99.* © 1993-1998 Microsoft
     Corporation. All rights reserved.
50   Online Medical Dictionary
51   Online Medical Dictionary

The Impulse-Control Disorders Not Elsewhere Classified contains behavioral disorders such as explosive anger, stealing, setting fires, gambling and pulling out one's hair. Some mental illnesses include these symptoms. Mania, for example, contains explosive anger while schizophrenia contains the hair behavior.

The Adjustment Disorders are maladaptive reactions to identifiable psychosocial stressors occurring within a short time after onset of a stressor. They are manifested by either impairment in social or occupational functioning or by symptoms (depression, anxiety, etc.) that are in excess of a normal and expected reaction to a stressor.[52]

The Personality Disorders are: Paranoid Personality, Schizoid Personality, Schizotypal Personality, Antisocial Personality, Borderline Personality, Histrionic Personality, Narcissistic Personality, Avoidant Personality, Dependent Personality, Obsessive-Compulsive Personality and truly scientific one, Personality Disorder Not Otherwise Specified.

The thirteenth category is called "Other Conditions That May Be a Focus of Clinical Attention".

Treatment

Once a diagnosis is made, treatment begins. Treatment is always a combination of drugs and counseling.

Drugs

Psychiatrists prescribe drugs from a quiver thirty-eight.

Schizophrenics and psychotics are incapable of representing themselves and, thus, have no choice: they must accept the drug regimen prescribed by their psychiatrists. Antipsychotic drugs, also called "Neuroleptics", are used to contain schizophrenia and psychosis.

---

52   On Line Medical Dictionary

Unipolars and Bipolars, however, are, following stabilization, capable of sharing responsibility for their drug course with their psychiatrists. These are the recent research indications for affective illness drug therapy:

(1) Unless treated very early in its eruption, your illness is will most likely continue to evolve.

(2) Drugs that are effective in one stage of your illness evolution can be completely ineffective in another.

(3) Your phenomenal brain creates its own drug-like reactions to your various illness expressions. Thus, your total "drug course" is a combination of the drug-like chemicals that your brain creates, plus those that you add from the outside. It is also suspected that exogenous (outside) drugs require endogenous (inside) drugs to react.[53]

(4) Therefore, when your illness evolution outgrows the effectiveness of your original drug course *do not* discontinue your original drugs. If you do, you will disrupt smoothly flowing chemical interactions and greatly diminish the effectiveness of any new outside drug. Rather, *add* new drugs to your original drugs.[54]

Combinations of antimanic and antidepressant drugs are often prescribed for bipolar illness. As described elsewhere, the process for finding the right drugs and combination of drugs is one of trial and error. Your goal in deciding upon the right drug and/or combination of drugs should not be perfect stabilization. It is my experience, not only in my own case, but also from my many observations over nineteen years, that no bipolar is perfectly stabilized. A better goal might be "almost stabilization".

---

53   Post, R.M., Denicoff, K.D., Frye, M.A., Dunn, R.T., Leverich, C.S., Osuch, E., Speer, A. 1998. A history of the use of anticonvulsants as mood stabilizers in the last two decades of the 20th century. *Neuropsycobiplogy Oct; 38(3)*: 152-66.

54   Weiss, S.R.B. & Post, R.M. 1998. Kindling: Separate vs. shared mechanisms in affective disorders and epilepsy. *Neuropsychobiology 38*: 167-180

The lesser mental disorders such a panic attacks and phobias are sometimes treated with antianxiety drugs. Antianxiety drugs are sometimes called "minor tranquilizers", as opposed to the "major tranquilizers", the neuroleptic drugs which are used to control schizophrenia.

Counseling

In addition to making a diagnosis made from 297 disorders, and prescribing a drug therapy chosen from 38 common psychotherapeutic drugs, the psychiatrists must now select one or more of 250 counseling therapies,[55] although the major ones number only four–psychoanalysis, behaviorism, cognitive and client-centered. Psychoanalysis has already been discussed, and the other three will be discussed in detail in the next chapter.

For a vast majority of mentally ill persons, counseling means individual and/or group therapy. Sometimes it includes family therapy. Individual therapy is best for crisis intervention and short-term problem solving. Group therapy, in which a number of patients gather to discuss their problems under the leadership of therapists, is best for long-term adjustment. In group therapy, the newly arrived have the opportunity to learn that they are not alone in their suffering and that there is life after mental illness. Group therapy costs far less than individual therapy.

In their befuddlement, however, most mentally ill persons do not stay on their drugs and do not continue therapy. Just as teenagers must rebel against their parents, the newly fledged mentally ill must rebel against their physicians, their drugs and their therapy.

It was true for me, and I believe that I have seen it in others, that respect for the therapy process begins only after hitting bottom. At that

---

55   "Psychotherapy," *Microsoft® Encarta® Encyclopedia 99.* © 1993-1998 Microsoft Corporation. All rights reserved.

point, survivors form an attitude something like, "I will not get well until I admit that I am sick".

Issues in Psychiatry

Trial and Error Diagnoses

Tales of incorrect diagnoses abound among psychiatric patients.

When I finally admitted that something was desperately wrong in my head and presented myself to a psychiatrist, I appeared to be a typical case of situational depression. My wife of twenty years had fallen in love with a neighbor.

In truth, I was either in a depressive swing of bipolar disorder or in the grips of Monroe's Episodic Disorder, either of which could have erupted, in accordance with my genetic and environmental inheritances, upon the discovery of my wife's betrayal.

The psychiatrist prescribed the antidepressant drug, *Elavil*. Unknown at the time (because neurologists had yet to discover the fact), the tricyclic antidepressant drugs have the side effect of inducing mania. Off I went into a mixed state of mania and depression, greatly complicating my life at a very critical time. The same psychiatrist, for whom I have the greatest admiration, eventually took me off *Elavil* and put me onto *lithium carbonate*, the only drug then available for bipolar disorder.

Almost every mentally ill person I know has a similar story. When *Thorazine* became available, almost every seriously ill patient was given that drug. I have been told that mental wards looked like morgues, with all the patients deeply asleep, whether in beds or chairs, or on floors or lawns. The same was true for *lithium carbonate*. Whether it worked for you or not, you got it because RESEARCH said it would.

Unfortunately, diagnosis is, and has been since the drug era began, a trial and error process even for the very best psychiatrists. I find myself wondering how Kraepelin would prescribe the new drugs, were he alive today. Would he ignore his initial impression of the patient and prescribe only after careful observation of his / her behavior? Or would he, feeling inclined to give immediate help, guess a diagnosis from initial impression and prescribe a drug on the first visit?

Whatever Kraepelin would do, modern psychiatrists do it on the first visit, and because the first drug prescribed often doesn't work well, those of us on the receiving end often feel that we are being experimented upon. In many instances we are. I have heard it said, "If the drug works, that's the diagnosis".

There are many reasons for prescribing drugs fast, money and suffering being first among them. Lots of visits to an office or lots of time in a hospital add up to big bucks at a time when the mentally ill are being crushed with anguish. The patient wants immediate help. The psychiatrist wants to give it. Who can fault him or her?

But one big reason for prescribing the old fashioned Kraepelin way is that while the right drug (or combination) is being found, the patient's brain/mind is afire with scary, uncontrollable thoughts and emotions, almost all of them faulty. If the drug of choice doesn't work quickly, he/she often stops taking it, turning on the psychiatrist for adding to her/his misery. The psychiatrist, in turn, throws up her/his hands and labels the patient "Non-compliant".

Not Listening to Patient Complaints

From 1970, when it became available in the United States, until 1995, when valproic acid replaced it as the drug of choice for mood control, *lithium carbonate* was prescribed to everyone suspected of having mania. Never mind that half their patients were telling their doctors that lithium didn't work, or that those patients simply stopped taking the drug because it obviously didn't work for them. "Research" convinced their physicians that lithium levels maintained at a careful level between toxicity and insufficiency "contained mania". If the patients said otherwise and balked at taking the drug, the patient was being non-compliant. That was just part of the frustration of being a psychiatrist.

For fourteen years, I lived (barely) with such nonsense. Then, God Bless him forever, Dr. Robert M. Post and his colleagues at the National Institute of Health published a paper showing that, while *lithium carbonate* is a wonderful drug for about 50% of bipolars, it ranges in effectiveness from barely to not-at-all for the other 50%.[56] In 1995, I was switched from *lithium carbonate* to *valproic acid*, and the relief that I experienced was profound.

Once again, I do not fault the psychiatrists who, for fourteen years, kept giving lithium to me, for they had nothing else to prescribe; and had I been they, I would also have felt a need to do something. What is irritating to the core, however, was their universal rejection that I might have been complaining in reality, not in illusion. They consider me, after all, "bipolar", not schizophrenic; and I am mentally ill, not mentally retarded.

From my point of view, this sort of "one size fits all" drug treatment is not so different from the spinning chairs that were once used to treat depression, the "tranquilizing (restraining) chair" that was used to treat mania, or the use of punishments and bleedings.

Lack of Experience on Both Sides of the Couch

Psychiatrists have abundant training experiences and no end of observations of mental illness from outside of the illnesses, but they have no first hand knowledge of what it feels like inside a mental illness. Because *every* human's perceptions are formed through the filter of her or his emotions, this lack of true understanding of the inside experience

---

56   Post, R.M.; Ketter, T.A.; Pazzaglia, P.J.; Denicoff, K.; George, M. S.; Callahan, A.; Leverich, G.; Fry, M., (1996). Rational polypharmacy in the bipolar affective disorders. *Epilepsy-Res-Suppl., 11:* 153-80.

is obvious to the mentally ill, and is a source of doubt in our psychiatrists that can lead to disrespect.

What is required is acknowledgement by both parties that two experts face each other in therapy, one with outside experiences and one with inside experiences. It often happens, however, that one or both denies the expertness of the other and therapy fails.

The Endless Knot

From this Underview of the psychiatric diagnosis and treatment process, two things are, I hope, evident: That psychiatry is a very complex, often imperfect undertaking, and that the interactions of health-seeker and health-giver are likewise very complex.

The psychiatrist, of course, has the advantage, not least because he or she is in command of their emotions. The mentally ill, however, arrive in the office of the psychiatrist in states ranging from outright denial that they are ill to despair that they will ever get well. In between these black and white bookends are thousands of shades of gray complicated with faulty thoughts and emotions, some generated by the illness ("Everything is coming apart!"), and some generated in reaction to the illness ("Why me?"). The psychiatrist must see through them all to their root cause and decide upon a course of treatment, which is sort of like seeing past the surface of a lake into its depths. The best psychiatrist, therefore, is a highly empathetic, careful scientist. To some, that will sound like an oxymoron. But they do exist, to my certain knowledge.

4

Clinical Psychology

"Psyche" is Greek for "soul", which today we call "mind", so Psychology is literally the study of the soul/mind. Psychology as philosophy began with the ancient Greeks and it remained in the realm of philosophy until the emergence, at the same time, of Sigmund Freud's Psychoanalysis and Ivan Pavlov's Classical Conditioning. From that point in history, Psychology blossomed into a scientific discipline.

The Training and Functions of Psychologists

Psychologists receive a "Doctor of Philosophy" (Ph.D.) degree after attaining a four year Bachelors degree and a Masters degree. The Ph.D. degree is received after completion of a doctoral dissertation based upon research and conclusions acceptable to the graduate school awarding the degree. The amount of time required to achieve a Ph.D. varies greatly, but it would be a rare genius that could complete one in less than six years. There is also a "Clinical Psychology" degree (Psy.D.) that does not include the research component.

Psychology has numerous areas of specialized study ranging from rigorous experimental technique to armchair theorizing. In practice, clinical and counseling psychologists treat the mentally ill and they apply an eclectic "basket of therapies" to each patient based upon need. For example, the same patient might need the emotive encouragement of client-centered therapy, the thinking clarification of cognitive therapy, and the organizational structure of behavioral therapy all at the same time.

Three Major Psychologies

Behaviorism

In 1904, while studying nerve reactions in dogs, Ivan Pavlov, a Nobel laureate, discovered by accident what others came to call "Classical Conditioning". In its simplest definition, Classical Conditioning is a form of neuronal learning in which a response transfers from one stimulus to another. The story that I related above of me confusing my father's dirty fingernails with those of workers in a plant is an example of a transferred response from one stimulus to another. While many psychologists would discount my fingernail example as an example of Classical Conditioning because the two stimuli occurred over a great passage of time, I am convinced from personal experience that confusion of long and short-term memory is a major component of my mental illness.

Following his discovery, Pavlov spent more than three decades studying the processes underlying classical conditioning. He and his associates identified four main processes: acquisition (initial learning), extinction (elimination of the conditioning), generalization (response to similar stimuli without additional training), and discrimination (the opposite of discrimination).

Today, psychologists use classical conditioning to explain some cases of phobias, which are irrational or excessive fears of specific objects or situations. A person who receives only bills and letters from debt collectors in her mailbox may develop a phobia against opening her mail. Such a phobia is not a serious mental illness, and the concepts of classical conditioning may very well be used to treat such a reaction.

Classical conditioning also partially explains the behavior of neurons and neuronal pathways in the body and the brain. A cascade of neuron behavior perhaps explains the process by which a person jerks his finger (response) off a hot burner (stimulus).

In 1913, Edward L. Thorndike built upon the Pavlov results by developing what he called the "law of effect". In summary, this "law" states the intuitively obvious: That behaviors followed by pleasant consequences (like candy) will be strengthened, and that behaviors followed by unpleasant consequences (like spankings) will be weakened.

At about the same time, the American psychologist John B. Watson began developing his science of "Behaviorism". Watson did not perceive Freud's psychology of exploring and correcting inner experiences or feelings by subjective, introspective methods to be a true science. Watson did not deny the existence of inner experiences, but he held that such experiences could not be studied and reproduced by other scientists because they were not observable. Greatly influenced by Pavlov's work, Watson proposed to make the study of psychology scientific by using only objective procedures, such as laboratory experiments designed to establish statistically significant results. This behaviorist view led him to proclaim that emotional reactions are learned in much the same way as other skills. Watson's stimulus-response theory resulted in a tremendous increase in research activity on learning in animals and in humans, from infancy to early adulthood.[57]

In the 1930's, B. F. Skinner further developed the ideas of Pavlov, Thorndike and Watson into a science that he called "Operant Conditioning", which he claimed could explain how rewards and punishments control the majority of human behavior. So far, Skinner's claim has not been supported by the evidence.

57　"Behaviorism," *Microsoft® Encarta® Encyclopedia 99.* © 1993-1998 Microsoft Corporation. All rights reserved.

Today, Behaviorism is most useful to Behavioral Psychologists who treat the mentally retarded and severely mentally ill. Teaching self-care skills to schizophrenics and reducing their aggressive and antisocial behaviors can be accomplished with Operant Conditioning. It is useful in treating stuttering, sexual disorders, drug additions, impulsive disorders, and eating disorders. It is also quite helpful in explaining how serious mental illness flowers out of genetic inheritance and childhood trauma, reinforced intermittently just as Pavlov's dogs were. Recall the Post Model of Affective Illness discussed above and note how much Behaviorism is evident in the model:

1. A genetic weakness, which results in faulty amygdala functioning, appears to exist.

2. Childhood and adolescent traumas (in those with the genetic weakness) proceed bipolar disorder eruption and "train" [**Behaviorism**] neuronal pathways in the brain/mind for later illness-inducing stress.

3. A first eruption of bipolar disorder, or "kindling", succeeds or fails in direct relationship to the quality of previous traumatic memories and neuronal pathway training [**Behaviorism**]. Thus, childhood and adolescent traumas are the parents of bipolar disorder eruption.

4. A kindling event alone will not flame into self-sustaining bipolar disorder. For that to happen, a kindling event must be subsequently reinforced in an intermittent way in accordance with the discoveries of Pavlov, Thorndike, Watson and Skinner [**Behaviorism**].

5. Lacking intervention with drug and counseling therapies, bipolar disorder eruption graduates from a psychosocial reaction stage (with reinforcement) [**Behaviorism**] into a stage of internal genesis in which "episodes begat episodes"

[**Behaviorism**]. At this point, the illness becomes automatic and uncontrollable [**Behaviorism**].

Note, however, that behaviorism does not explain the entire Post Model. Genes, environment and a faulty amygdala are required in addition to Behaviorism's intermittent reinforcement and nerve "training". Clearly, though, the science of behaviorism explains a lot. Like everything else, however, it is only a part, not all, of the answer to mental illness. I, for one, do not think behaviorism can answer this question: How does your science explain the random behaviors of a person with a faulty amygdala?

Cognitive Therapy

Just as behavioral therapies are built upon the idea of changing behaviors, cognitive therapies are built upon the ideas of changing beliefs and thoughts. A major difference between them, however, is that behavioral therapies are built upon hard science (that is, objective measurement of change) while cognitive therapies are built upon soft science (that is, subjective measurement of change).

This approach began to take form in the 1950's when psychologist Albert Ellis developed *rational-emotive therapy* now commonly called *rational-emotive behavior therapy*. Ellis was a practicing psychoanalysis until, in the 1940s, he became disillusioned with Freud's methods, viewing them as slow and inefficient.

Influenced by Alfred Alder's work, Ellis came to regard irrational beliefs and illogical thinking as the major cause of most emotional disturbances. Negative *events* such as losing a job or breaking up with a lover do not by themselves cause depression or anxiety. Rather, a person's *reactions* to such events (such as by thinking, "I'm a worthless human being") cause the depression and anxiety.

The most common technique of rational-emotive behavior therapists is to dispute (what the therapist perceives to be) irrational thoughts.

First the therapist identifies irrational beliefs by talking with the client about his or her problems. Examples of irrational beliefs might include the idea that unhappiness is caused by external events, that one must be accepted and loved by everyone, that one must always be competent and successful to be a worthwhile person.[58]

The weakness in this therapy that I perceive is the usual one–that the therapists assumes the position of "perfect mind" and puts the patient in the position of "imperfect mind", when, in truth, the patient's problem may very well be a biological problem, not a thinking problem.

In the 1960's, Aaron T. Beck also became disenchanted with Freudian Psychoanalysis and embraced Ellis' ideas. Beck is now the best known cognitive therapist. He has published many books, and his *Beck Depression Inventory*, a device for measuring the severity of depression, is widely used.

Client-Centered Therapy

In 1957, Carl R. Rogers published his hypothesis of constructive personality change. This is the therapy that has been most helpful to me.

His core argument is that the mentally ill have the capacity to understand and change their self-concepts, attitudes, and self-directed behaviors, and that these resources can be unleashed by certain *therapist behaviors.*[59]

There are three parts to his "therapist behaviors", presented simply here:

---

58 "Psychotherapy," *Microsoft® Encarta® Encyclopedia 99.* © 1993-1998 Microsoft Corporation. All rights reserved.

59 Brodley, B.T., (1986) "Client-Centered Therapy–What Is It? What Is It Not?", paper presented at the Association for the Development of Person-Centered Approach, University of Chicago, September 3-7.

1. The more genuine, and less "professional" the therapists is, the greater the likelihood that the client will change and grow in a constructive manner.

2. When the therapist maintains a positive, nonjudgmental, non-directed, accepting attitude toward the client, therapeutic change is more likely.

3. Empathic understandings, based upon sensing the personal meaning of a client's thoughts and feelings, "re-framing" them and returning them with acceptance, hastens healing.

Note the difference between Freud and Rogers. With Freud, the relationship of therapist and client are inherently unequal. The client is defined as vulnerable and in need of help while the therapist is defined as invulnerable and all knowing. With Rogers, client and therapist are equal. Authority is shared. The final interpretation of the client's experiences and the way the client uses the therapeutic relationship is entrusted to the client.

Rogers' psychology was, of course, developed before the biopsychiatric revolution–back when there was no hard science explanation of mental illness, when observation and not a little personal philosophy went into the development of mental illness therapies. Today, a great deal of neurological research indicates that at least bipolar disorder is an organic illness of the brain, new knowledge that calls into question whether a person with bipolar disorder can permanently change "self-directed behaviors".

Even so, with the single reservation that it worked slowly (it may be more accurate to say that *I* worked slowly), I found Client-Centered Therapy far more effective than the other therapies that I encountered. I envision my breakeven process like this: it took me fourteen years to get on the right drugs for me; once my moods were stabilized, I began to construct a scaffold of a new mind around my old mind. It was in the constructing of my new scaffold that Client-Centered Therapy was extremely helpful.

The Complexities of Counseling

While biological psychiatry focuses on the inner problems of neuronal "misbehavior", the science of psychology focuses on helping the whole person make it in the normal world.

Psychosis ("the state of being out of touch with reality") is a recurring problem in severe mental illness, and those suffering the illness cannot heal themselves or even approach a "normal" life without considerable outside help. A sympathetic, reality-based mind is needed, against which the sufferer may compare his or her own psychotic thoughts and feelings. Even for the lucky psychotics that do not lose their support systems, trained counselors are essential to the reality-check function.

Counseling is not easy. No two cases of BPI, for example, are exactly the same. Counseling can be thankless. Commitments made in either mania or depression can be forgotten when in the other state. Irritation and anger are prominent emotions in bipolar disorder; sometimes they are directed at counselors. In rapid cycling bipolar disorder, confusion predominates and counseling becomes akin to King Canute commanding the tide not to rise.

Here is an example.

As previously mentioned, I carry the diagnosis of "Bipolar II". I am uncertain of the science behind that diagnosis and suspect that my experiences are better categorized by Kraepelin's generic diagnosis of "Manic-Depression". Whichever is the more correct terminology, these were my experiences before taking *valproic acid*.

I had about four times as much depression as mania (as measured by charts that I kept on myself). Most of my depression was profound, meaning suicidal. Most of my mania was mild, meaning that I had happy, forceful energy surges that included delusions and hallucinations.

In the depressed state, time became slippery for me and I drifted along in it like a leaf in a stream. Things mental would not stay put, I could not recall recipes, computer commands, well-known telephone numbers, appointments, nor obligations. I had no wit, no ideas, no interest in sex, and almost no physical or mental energy. I felt angry about things that I couldn't identify. I felt that people (friends, strangers, it mattered not) were pulling back, mystified by me, frightened of me, concerned for me, exasperated with me. I suspected that they could peer into my mind and were revolted by what they saw. I felt as if my skin was running down my body like candle wax, and that people who noticed were revolted. They seemed to talk about things that I could not remember happening, they mentioned grand ideas (my own) that sounded foolish. I would try to hide from them hoping to regroup, to "pull things together", but I plunged, instead, even lower, completely disoriented by what was happening.

At its worst, I hallucinated a multi-tentacled misery sucking at my "real mind". I was terrified. I felt that it was stealing my mind, and that I was powerless to stop it. Because it returned over and over, it was the bane of my existence. It had no people in it, no devils, no briars, no heat nor cold, neither up nor down, no light, no odors, and no touches, nothing except flawless, never-ending emptiness and excruciating pain. I couldn't fight it. I was like a wasp that had been poisoned by a spider, alive, but totally numb. People on the outside of me were merciless. "Snap out of it," "pull yourself together," "everybody gets the blues". BANG, BANG, BANG, the insults kept coming. I tried to hide from them, regroup and re-engage when I was "real". But "realness" and relief never seemed to come, and I began to feel that I must kill my body in order to kill the pain. I tried six times.

That was depression.

Michael Crawford

Here is mania: My clock raced and my energy, sexual, physical and mental, soared. My ideas erupted like fireworks and I became groovy with people. Words flooded out of me, written words, spoken words, jokes, wit and songs. I had (what I believe to be) incredible power to weave my words and emotions into a sort of music that made me (and others, so I believed) very happy. When asked if it were difficult to write his music, J.S. Bach replied, "Nothing to it, you just put the right note in the right place at the right time". That was me when I was high, just the right word at just the right place at just the right time. I was quick, too, quicker than just about anyone. I anticipated words before others could think of what to say. When I sold textbooks for an educational publisher, I often gave one-hour sales presentations to buyers who never got to say a word; in their behalf, I even posed questions to myself, which I then answered brilliantly, of course. I could do such things because, when high, I was incredibly sensitive to others. From body language, words, expression, who knows what else, I (believed that I) could "read" the feelings, desires, fears and regrets of others like chapters in a book. People invited me to become involved with them (it may have been the reverse), and I did, in tender ways, in outraged ways, but never in passive ways. My sexual fantasies were limitless. Beautiful music aroused me. Verse aroused me. Nature aroused me. I sometimes imagined myself as a tree being pollinated. Once I felt like a bee having intercourse with flowers. An especially erotic image was molten gold squirting from the magma up into granite faults at the Earth's surface. Once in the mountains I envisioned metamorphic rock being folded under the surface of the earth by God, where he heated it, pressed it, and returned it to the surface, transformed into gneiss. At such times, I could never get enough sex. After sex, I masturbated. In my giddiness, I thought of myself as possessing special powers, of intelligence, insight, understanding and explanation. No idea was too big. I felt that I had a special relationship with God. I thought I could write like Shakespeare, Dostoevski, Kazantzakis, Tolkien; or identify all the sacred literature published since the Bible; or explain how neutrons connect us to the Universe. But though I clearly understand how to do such things, I started none, because I skipped from idea to idea like lightening in a thunderstorm. Believe it or not, I was never aware when I was in the manic state. It fooled me every time because I considered it to be the "real me".

My highs never lasted. They were always too brief. At some point in the wonderful mood, sleep disturbances would begin. Some seemed more real than real. They awakened me with a start, my heart pounding, telephones ringing, loud words spoken as if from God, my daughter crying "Daddy!" I once heard an orchestra playing the first note of Hyden's Surprise Symphony. Sometimes I saw colors mixing as if a rainbow were spilling on the ground. I was once scared witless by a large bird that flew beneath my covers and attacked me with its sharply pointed bill; that time, I bounded from bed and shut myself in the bathroom.

My mental speed became like the crest of a wave that goes faster than its base, suddenly, I would find myself hovering over a precipice. Where has my friends and co-workers gone? They were lagging. They were looking at me in funny ways. I grew irritated. Very irritated. After all that I have done for them, they were standing back and letting me do all the work. To heck with them! I would do all the work! I would show them!

Suddenly, without warning, my anger erupted like Mount Saint Helen. I never became physically violent, but I did switch to sharp words and an angry tone. Emotionally, I blew everyone away. Things fell apart and back into depression I would go.

Very few marriages can withstand such behavior. Even mothers give up on it. Even empathetic psychologists do when patients stop taking their drugs.

5

A Case History That Supports the Post Model of Affective Illness

This case history is about me. But before I present it, I would like to make a few stipulations.

First, writing clearly about mental illness is greatly complicated by the fact that only a small part of our understanding of it is based upon hard science. The Kindling Effect of Goddard, *ET Al,* is good, objective, hard science. On the other hand, whether bipolar disorder is a "Mood Disorder" or a "Psychosis" is pure subjective soft science. At its best, the Bible of clinical psychiatry, the DSM-IV, from which my diagnosis comes, is a library of mental illness philosophy, arrived at not in a laboratory but in a committee room. Therefore, I cannot write with certainty that I am a Bipolar II. As I established earlier, Russell Monroe's diagnosis, "Episodic Disorder", far more accurately describes the mental illness that I experience. Yet the psychiatric industry has labeled me a "Bipolar II", and that brand has gained wide acceptance; so, to communicate clearly, I will, in what follows, call myself a "Bipolar II" and abbreviate my illness "BPII".

With that cravat allowed for, let us now turn to "The Post Model of Affective Illness". Please note that this model is presented as my own understanding of the work of Dr. Post and many others. I do not claim to present Post's own opinions. I very much hope that I do not misrepresent him in any way.

I perceive the Post Model to have seven steps, and this case study is presented that way.

Step One: Genes and Childhood Environment

My Maternal Grandfather

My maternal grandfather, "Daddy Ray", whom I lived next to and whom I adored, belonged to the seventh generation of his family in America. His ancestors, Scots-Irish clockmakers from Londonderry, arrived in Yorktown, Virginia, on a William Byrd ship. They fought the Revolutionary War at the Battle of Yorktown, where they lived. After the war, they moved into the interior of the continent, first to Frederick County, Virginia, then across the Blue Ridge Mountains to Ireland, Virginia, in that part of the state that eventually became West Virginia. They stayed there as stanch Unionist for the duration of the Civil War, then moved west again, to the rich black prairie of Illinois, where they bought a farm in Carthage, a town near the Mississippi. That farm is still in the Clark family.

The town next to Carthage is Nauvoo, where Joseph Smith and his Mormons settled. The Clarks were there when the Mormons arrived, and, according to Daddy Ray, they didn't like the Mormon's polygamy any more than did the easterners. At some point, Joe Smith was arrested and put into the Carthage jail. One night, he was sent to draw water from the well. A group of locals were waiting and gunned him down. Shortly thereafter, the Mormons departed for Utah, and Daddy Ray, his parents and a paternal uncle, departed for Houston. Was there a connection between the two events? Daddy Ray never said that there was; but Philip Clark, the owner of the farm in 1984, told me that family legend held that a Clark was part of the murder.

Once in Houston, the Clarks purchased and farmed land on the north side of the city. Soon after their arrival, and while he was still a boy, both of Daddy Ray's parents died, leaving him to be reared by his paternal uncle, "Uncle Bob". I have a single memory of Uncle Bob. He arrived one morning at Daddy Ray's front door, a tall slim man dressed in a dark suit, white shirt, bow tie and a black cane with a metal tip. He had come, he explained, to teach trigonometry to my brother and me who, at the time, were in elementary school. He called us to my grandfather's dinning room table, a massive Victorian piece of oak (upon which my grandmother had delivered all her children), and proceeded to instruct us verbally, punctuated by impatient stamps of his cane upon the wooden floor. Neither my brother nor I could understand his instructions and soon there were more stamps of his cane than words. He sent me away first. I knew when he was finished with my brother by his cane tapping, which had begun to sound like a machine gun. He walked out of the house shouting words that I couldn't understand. That night, Daddy Ray asked me what I thought of Uncle Bob. I told him that he tapped his cane a lot. Daddy Ray smiled and said no more.

When his parents died, stern old Uncle Bob reared Daddy Ray, taking for wife a stern old daughter from the farm next door. He had fallen in love with Lila Jones, a sweet and loving soul. But when he asked farmer Jones for Lila's hand, Uncle Bob was told that the older daughter, Lena, had to marry first. So Uncle Bob married Lena and took both sisters into his home, where they formed a three-way relationship that lasted until their deaths. Lena managed the family finances with brilliance, and Lila loved Uncle Bob. For those of you who don't recognize this story, it is an eerie echo from the first book of the Bible, Genesis, Chapter 29, the story of Jacob, Rachel and Leah.

It wasn't until after Daddy Ray's death that I learned what happened next. Daddy Ray couldn't stand his new mother, so he ran away, lied about his age and joined the Navy. On his first cruise, he deserted somewhere near Corpus Christi, Texas. He returned to Houston and went to work for Blackshear's Market in the Fifth Ward of Houston. The Fifth Ward had been developed to house railroad workers. At the time, Houston had seventeen railroads, the largest of which was the Southern Pacific. One fateful day, when Daddy Ray was delivering groceries in a horse-drawn wagon, he spotted Dorothy Haver on her front porch, and the love-starved young man found the partner that would last his lifetime.

Daddy Ray and Arkie (as "Dorothy" somehow came to be called) married and had four children. He supported them by working first as a policeman, then as the clerk of the District (State) Court in Houston. By the time I became aware of things, they also had three grandchildren. That number would later grow to eleven. On weekends, Daddy Ray's family of seventeen, joined by my grandmother's two sisters, two brothers and occasional members of their families would gather under the hickory tree in the back yard for family get-togethers that came to be called, "Arkieville". Daddy Ray, who taught himself to play every stringed instrument, including a twelve-stringed guitar, provided most of the entertainment.

It seemed so happy to me. Yet, Daddy Ray was a depressed man. Perhaps because he perceived that he was unloved as a child; perhaps because he never finished high school; perhaps because he deserted from the Navy; perhaps because his depression was not situational at all, but caused by faulty brain chemistry, Daddy Ray was a depressed man. And because I absolutely adored the man, I was probably imprinted with how "to do" depression.

My Maternal Grandmother

My grandmother, Arkie, was absolutely unique. She laughed and sang all day and never had downs or low energy. If I did not wake up early enough, Arkie would make my bed with me still in it, all the while singing a song about sleepy-heads or pretending to be perplexed by the "lump" in the bed. Whatever the time of day, she would stop what she was doing and cook whatever I wanted to eat, which was, most often, "white" pan cakes, as opposed to the yellow ones (made from corn meal) that Daddy Ray preferred. I often shopped with her, walking to and from the market with fish-net bags that Daddy Ray wove for her. Once she promised me a "present" for going with her. At the market, I was unable to choose a toy. When we got home, however, I decided. Without a word of protest, she walked me back.

She had a very English face, meaning a prominent nose on a basically flat face. Her mouth was about half the size of Daddy Ray's, but it smiled just as much. She had long auburn hair which she wore sometimes as a bun on the back of her head, but most often as a crown. Her bosom was larger than huge and very intimidating, I had to plan how to hug her so that I would not be suffocated. Daddy Ray liked to sit with an arm around her, his broad hand resting on the side of a breast; even so, his hand covered only half. She had a strong soprano voice that could take over an entire church of voices. Often I would hear her whisper, "Ray, they are singing too slow." Daddy Ray would say, "OK". Together, they would raise their voices and speed up the entire congregation, Arkie's voice dominant and sweet like icing on a cake.

Arkie was the magnet who held the family together. It was she that the relatives came to see on weekends. After she died, the weekend get-togethers ceased. I was amazed. I thought everyone came to see Daddy Ray.

Arkie was fifth generation Haver. Edward Hodgson Haver (1860-1944), his wife, Alice Crease (1866-1944), and three children immigrated to Houston from Newcastle Upon Tyne, England, to take a job making tools and dies for the Southern Pacific Railroad. Two more children were born in Houston, one of them Arkie (1893-1963).

The line started when Justice Haver (1752-1830) emigrated from Hesse Cassel, Germany, to Ponteland, England, and married Elizabeth Smith (1787-?). The family lived in Newburn and Newcastle Upon Tyne until Edward moved his family to Houston. I remember three often discussed anecdotes about Edward. First, he invented a pecan-sheller for which he never got paid. "They" stole it from him, although none of my family knew who "they" were. Secondly, he belonged, in England and in Houston, to an organization that believed in mental telepathy. Conan Doyle, the author of Sherlock Holmes, was a member. Edward would arrange by mail, with members of the organization still in England, to think about a particular shape at a certain time on a certain day. The English and American experimenters would then correspond to learn if "communication" had occurred. I tried to track down such mail, but could find none. Thirdly, Edward had the curious habit of disappearing whenever his wife, called "Bobo," got pregnant. After the child was born, Edward would return and Bobo would take him back. They never moved from their house on Mercer Street, so I can only guess that he provided money for her; he had a good job. There were no anecdotes to explain why Edward withheld his emotional support, so my memory of him is fuzzy. However, I do think it possible, from these family anecdotes, to suspect that my mother's grandfather was mechanically gifted and emotionally unstable.

My memory of Bobo is likewise fuzzy, the strongest of which being of her sitting on the front porch of Arkie's house, frail and white and dressed in black. I was afraid of her, though I can not remember why. My mother loved her as much as I did Daddy Ray, and had a life-long fear that she "would be treated like Bobo." Later, I figured out that what mother feared was being shunted, as Bobo had been, between the homes of her children after her husband died. Bobo was cared for that way because she had something wrong topside, as revealed by this anecdote about her daily behavior while staying with Arkie. Every day, she would gather unattached items from the rooms of the house and put them on the dining room table; then, as my uncles and Daddy Ray returned from school and work, they would collect their things from the table and return them to their rightful places. Bobo could not remember their names. She called my mother, "Sister" and each of my uncles, "Brother."

Such behaviors are often attributed to Alzheimer's Disease, and perhaps she had that problem; but, maybe not. My mother repeated Bobo's circular and obsessive behavior in her old age; yet, when we had her autopsied at death, she did not have Alzheimer's, she did not even have Profound Dementia...she had Normal Dementia. Before I came to be medicated with drugs that work for me, I, too, engaged in circular and obsessive behavior.

My Mother

To my early mind, my mother was like a skipping stone, but more complicated; she was more like a skipping stone seen through a kaleidoscope. The skips, splashes and circles that she made on still surfaces were fun to watch, and always colorful; but I never knew where she would go next, and, when she eventually stopped skipping, she sank into "The Blues". She loved all babies very much, but she loved me especially much, and the love was mutual. In fact, I adored her. One of my earliest memories is of sitting on the kitchen floor in Kilgore (I was a toddler), Mother with her back to me. She was washing something in the sink. Suddenly, a huge wind, cold with bluster, blew open the front and back doors with house-shaking bangs; the door of the oven crashed down in fury, and a baking pie therein jumped out. It rolled across the floor, a disk of flames, and away into oil fields behind our house.

I thought she had done it just for my enjoyment. I screamed with delight and laughed, hoping that she would do it again. But she never did. Later, when I could talk better, I often asked her how she did it, but she always pretended not to know what I was talking about; but then, she also pretended to have never washed out my mouth with soap for saying naughty words.

She was the best Rubber-Band-Pistol and Sling-Shot-Maker in the neighborhood. I achieved very high status with them. Whenever I shot a cousin or a friend with one, I usually took the victim home to ask my Wizard Mother to make another for them. Yes, she got mighty tired of making them, but she never said no and all my cousins and friends told me that I had the best mother in the world. But I knew that.

Oddly enough, my pride in my mother and my powerful feelings of special love between us were, I think, the source of early anxiety. Anxiety is the acid of mental illness. It oozes in sick minds and corrodes all mental activity. Textbooks define it as "an emotional fear response to a non-specific threat"; I had lots of such fear responses with my mother.

For example, when mother ignored me to hug and ooh and ahh over a new baby, I wondered if she were wishing for children other than her own. This caused me anxiety because alcoholism canceled-out my father as a source of emotional support. Skipping stone though she might be, she was, in my moments of emotional need, the most important parent I had.

Believe it or not, even her beauty gave me a chance to make anxiety. She was always happy when dressing. She had a large mouth that exploded with dazzling smiles. Her teeth were perfect and white, her cheekbones high, her eyes hazel, her hair short and brunette and her body slim. She "did" her face and fingernails and even her toenails. She always wore earrings and high-heeled shoes. She turned heads. She looked so young that my older brother's friends sometimes assumed her to be his sister, which she loved.

Money, of course, is the Mother's Milk of anxiety, and mother was like Johnny Appleseed with it. My father worked all week to earn a small amount of money, all of which, except for beer and gas money, he gave to Mom. By mid-week, it was all gone, sometimes spent well, sometimes not, sometimes "lent" to relatives in need. As a child, I dreaded paydays, which were every Friday night. Arguments between my parents over where the money had gone were loud and never ending. Until we learned to stay clear of them, my brother and I almost always got Friday-night spankings. My father, slurring his words, would fold his belt in two and call it his "double-licker". Spankings made me cry uncontrollably, not so much because they hurt my body, but because they made me feel extreme anxiety.

I often wondered, back then, how my Wizard Mother could love such a man. As I grew older, however, I figured it out. She liked beer, too. One evening, my two younger sisters came to me crying. They were frightened about mother, who was at Aunt Alice's house, in her driveway, laughing hysterically and ignoring their pleas to come home. I got on my bike and was there in two or three minutes. I found them drunk and howling with laughter. It took shouting and pulling on mother's arms to get her attention. It was humiliating. I knew that all the neighbors were listening. After a loud conversation, I was finally able to convince her that the girls and I were frightened by her behavior. When she finally came home, she professed amazement that she had frightened us. She promised to never drink again. At first she kept the promise; but as time went on, she broke it. Whenever she drank, my anxieties soared.

There is another emotional precursor in my early life, a tangential one that must be mentioned here. My mother was the oldest of four children, the three youngest being boys. The last one is my Uncle Terry, who spent, in the 40's and early 50's, a fair amount of time in the psychiatric ward of the Houston VA Hospital. He was there prior to the biopsychiatry revolution (no antidepressants, no *lithium*), when Freudian psychology was the treatment of choice for the mentally ill. Terry, who was color-blind as I am, sometimes went on wild spending sprees and drunken binges. His utilities were often turned off and he occasionally "borrowed" money from my mother, which never failed to make my father furious. My other two maternal uncles were very stable.

My Paternal Grandfather

My paternal grandfather was Marvin David Crawford, and I know a few things about him, but not much. He was born in Tallassee, Alabama and grew up in Arcadia, Louisiana. He married my grandmother, Nancy Caroline Pearce (1886-1961) on November 22, 1908. He bought a Model T kit from Henry Ford, rigged it with a saw on the back and drove his "saw mill" to building sites in the piney hills of northern Louisiana. On a street in Arcadia, Louisiana, he told my father's brother that a woman with an umbrella was a man with a Tommy Gun. In Longview, Texas, he took a relative's laundry delivery truck out on a rural road and left it there. He was committed to the State Mental Hospital in Pineville, Louisiana after my grandmother signed a certain paper. Her Pearce brothers took him there, apparently without resistance from any of his family. Marvin's half-brother, Henry, visited him in the hospital. Marvin was peaceful and making things with his hands (a form of therapy still in use today). Uncle Henry told me that some authority figure (his memory was vague), told him that "Marvin didn't belong there". Marvin eventually left the hospital (I do not know if he did so with or without permission), and was never seen again. A pair of new work boots was mysteriously left for my father at his Kilgore, Texas, home. My mother thought the boots were from Marvin. My father talked to me about him one time, when I was in college and he was about 48. As usual, he was sitting on the back steps, treating his "Blues" with beer. He said a few words of praise about his father, welled up with tears and said no more. My mother thought Marvin's behavior was understandable because my grandmother Crawford did not like sex.

That's it. Those are the few facts that I have been able to pry out of family members about my paternal grandfather Crawford. I have never tried to get his records from Pineville. Back then, in America, all mental illness was called Schizophrenia.

My Paternal Grandmother

We called my paternal grandmother "Nanny", and we children adored her. She was a full-sized woman with salt and pepper hair, which she wore as a knot on the back of her head. The triangle shape of her face very much resembled that of my father. She always dressed in black and rarely smiled, unless she was telling a Bible Story, which she did with great joy and drama. My parents were always tense when she visited. She believed that alcohol and tobacco were instruments of the Devil, and my father embraced them both. When television came, it, too, was an instrument of the Devil. To the best of my knowledge, she watched only a single telecast, of a Billy Graham revival.

Her arrivals were dramatic. Her old Nash that looked like an upside-down bathtub would roll into the driveway and a tense message would flow through the house like a bolt of electricity—"she's here!" Before we could go to her, she was in the house, herding us into the living room. There we would all kneel down and listen to her pray for us. I am not sure that I ever heard her words, but I felt her emotions loudly and they frightened me. When the prayers ended, however, she hugged and kissed us and was wonderful in every way.

My favorite story was that of Samson and Delilah, from the Book of Judges. Samson, of course, was a chosen of the Lord and, for a time, the champion of the Jews. In his time of acceptability to the Lord, he once killed a thousand Philistines with just the jawbone of an ass. But he fell from grace with God when he revealed to Delilah, a Philistine woman, that his God would give him strength only so long as he never cut his hair. Delilah promptly cut his hair and his enemies finally captured Samson. He was tied between the pillars of a temple in which the Philistine's celebrated their sweet victory over him. Samson then prayed to God to give him a final burst of strength so that he could pull down the house of the Philistines. The Lord did, and Nanny, playing the part of Samson, put out her arms as if they were bound to pillars, pulled a mighty pull, and brought down the temple upon Samson, the hated Philistines, my brother and me.

Much later, following my first hospitalization, when I was on *lithium carbonate* and in therapy, I had a recurring dream of myself as Superman, alive, but somehow framed as a picture in a corridor that held other pictures. My ex-wife arrived to look at me, holding a bottle of *lithium carbonate*. I collapsed and fell from the picture as if the drug were Kryptonite (i.e., the element that had the power to disabled the "real" Superman). With my Freudian therapist's help, I eventually traced the origins of my Superman dream to Nanny's story of Samson and Delilah. Believing my Bipolar highs to be a "strength," my unconscious mind perhaps rearranged multiple memories into a powerful, recurring and revealing dream of me as "Samson/Superman," *lithium carbonate* as "Shorn Hair/Kryptonite," and my ex-wife as "Herself/Delilah."

I know little about my grandmother's (Pearce) line. She was the daughter of James Wiley Pearce and Margaret Ann Lee. Margaret Ann Lee was born in Alabama in 1857, three years before the Civil War. I do not know how or where she met her husband, but I suspect that the two of them were part of the second or third-generation of Scot-Irish immigrants who left the East Coast and settled in the interior of the United States. I knew my grandmother's two brothers, "J.W." and Wiley, the two who took my Grandfather Crawford to the mental hospital, although, when I knew them, I did not know that they had done so. They were very big men, easily twice the size of my father. They had made money in the Kilgore oil field, though I do not know how much. My Houston family considered them rich. Perhaps they were. I remember them as lordly and demanding.

My Father

My father, David Everidge (1909-1984,) was, for the most part, an emotionally unavailable man. In the terminal phase of his life, he opened up and told me a lot about himself and his childhood; but during my youth, even when he "did" the Boy-Scouts with me, he was an emotionally reserved person, almost the opposite of Daddy Ray.

He was shorter than the Clark men were and when my brother David and I grew to full size, he was the shortest of all the men in his family. He had dark eyes in a face that was shaped like a triangle. He had his mother's somber mouth. He combed his jet-black hair straight back from his forehead. He liked to wear hats, real hats with brims that, when snapped down over his forehead, gave him a handsome, rakish look. He did not have an ounce of body fat. His favorite movie star was Gary Cooper, who played strong, silent types of men.

His school in Arcadia, Louisiana, was a single room for all grades. He was a favorite of its teacher, who picked him up each morning (in her one-horse carriage) and delivered him home each afternoon. Perhaps for that reason, he was a champion speller, the only one, to my knowledge, in the family. He was eight when his father was put away. I have often tried to imagine the occasion. Did he know it was going to happen, and did he have what must have been a prolonged and wrenching goodbye; or did he simply wake up one morning and learn that he would never see his father again? Either way, I suspect that the occasion was the defining event of his life. For the entire time of his life in which I knew him, he was chronically depressed. Always depressed, though, never high (except on alcohol). He was a good manager of money, something that manics never are.

Upon completion of the local school, my Grandmother Nanny sent him to a Methodist college in Kentucky, where, because neither drink nor smoke was allowed, he mixed like oil and water. He ran away, to where or for how long, I do not know. Somewhere on his adventure, however, in a boxcar with several others, he got into a fight with a hobo who was smoking a cigar. My father stopped the hobo's fist with his face and the hobo's lighted cigar with his nose. He returned home soon thereafter. Despite his mother's fondest hopes for him, he never achieved her level of piety. Back then a person had to choose between smoking and drinking and the (protestant) church. He chose smoking and drinking.

My father was the favorite of his Pearce uncles, and when they went west to the Kilgore, Texas, oil field, (in 1934) they took my father with them. He "roughnecked" for them, an oil patch term that means manual labor. At some point, the uncles put my father into the "Swabbing" business. Like cholesterol in a human body, goop from the East Texas oil would choke the pipes that brought it up, and "swabbers," like my father, would clean it out and haul it away for a fee. World War II broke out in 1939. With his family (my brother and I were born in Kilgore), he left the East Texas oil field and went to Houston, where mother would be near her family in case he was drafted. Then he found a job in a war-related industry, which kept him home from the battlefields. After the war was over, defense-related jobs disappeared and the vets came home. Jobs were scarce. Dad passed through his 20's when the nation passed through the Great Depression, and he was 36 when World War II ended. As a lot of people did, he emerged from that tumultuous time a very cautious person. He clung to the security of his blue-collar job like a child to his blanket. In his forties, the time of life when men come to grip with who they are, he watched the post-war boom pass him by, and his family grew by two daughters.

His life was also complicated by my mother's behavior. While my brother and I felt left out when our sisters came along, I suspect that Dad felt left out when my brother and I came along. Add Mother's spending habits and "The Blues" it seemed to give him, and I suppose that he had reason to drink. Daddy, too, was complex: high all weekend, but sober and responsible during the workweek.

Step Two: Major Childhood Anxiety Imprints

These anxiety imprints may appear pale to you. Compared to others that I have heard, they seem pale to me. It is not the strength or weakness of early anxiety imprints that matter, however. What matters is, as I understand the process, what a person's faulty amygdala does with those imprints. To extend the metaphor of William Wordworth's famous line of poetry, "The child is the father of the man", it might be said that "When the man, by chance, repeats the anxiety imprints of his childhood, his faulty amygdala confuses his adulthood anxiety with his childhood anxiety and possibly kindles into BPII".

(1) The Friday Night Rhythm

My father earned a modest paycheck and my mother gained self-esteem from spending it freely. This behavior led to a Friday Night Rhythm in which there was always a drunken argument over how the money had been and would be spent. Those loud and mutually recriminating arguments caused me pronounced feelings of worry for my mother and for myself. The rhythm always included a Friday Night Spanking, instigated by my big brother. I was terrified of the spankings that I knew would come as surely as the sunrise. But I was powerless to avoid them.

These repeated events predisposed my neuronal pathways for the emotion of anxiety.

(2) Two Homes, Two Sets of Parents

From ages three through twenty-one, I lived in two homes, one dysfunctional and one functional. The dysfunctional one was that of my parents. The functional one was that of my grandparents, next door.

Most often, I escaped the dysfunction of my parental home by burying myself in books. But when the dysfunction became unbearable, I escaped by going to my grandparent's home, where peace and bountiful love overflowed.

It is possible that this condition, repeated numberless times in random sequence, might have trained my neuronal pathways in the emotions of restlessness, agitation, avoidance and confusion.

(3) Lack of boundaries

My most bitter childhood memory is of Mother's raid on my penny collection. While in fourth grade I began collecting Lincoln Head pennies. With considerable effort I typed out a list of years and mints in which the pennies were minted, then struck off the year and mints as he added corresponding pennies to a jar. To protect the collection from my sisters, who were in kindergarten and second grade, and from whom nothing was safe, I hid the jar in my closet.

On the prodigiously happy day that I found the penny that completed my collection (when I was in sixth grade), I spread my pennies out, intending to arrange them by years and mints, only to discover that I didn't have the pennies that my list said I should. I flew into a rage against my sisters. My older brother, with whom I shared my room, might have pulled off the heist. But the culprits were much more likely to be my sisters. They were young and insatiably curious and mother enforced no boundaries whatsoever. Everyone's room and possessions were fair game for everyone else in the family. For those reasons, I suspected my sisters and asked Mother to avenge me.

Mother tried to put me off. For days, I demanded that she punish my sisters. But Mother responded with infuriating indirection—I could not pin her down to a punishment, but neither could I cease my angry attacks. I withdrew from my sisters, which hurt their feelings. They appealed to Mother to make me stop. At last, Mother admitted to me that she was the thief. On days when my sisters needed pennies with which to buy milk at school, and she had none to give, she borrowed from my penny jar. Then, when she had pennies to "repay" me, she put them back.

I was stupefied.

Mother knew that my pennies were a collection, not a slush fund. She had seen my list, contributed pennies to my collection, watched family members give me pennies from their pockets. She had often seen me spread out my collection on his bed and admire it.

In my memory, this was my first eruption of Jovian anger. I felt total rage towards Mother and tried to freeze her out of my life. I couldn't keep it up, of course. No child can function without a mother. But my relations with her were wary for the rest of my life. It is a measure of my anger that I carried it until I was fifty-two. As she lay on her deathbed, with all her children standing around her, telling her how much they loved her, I finally forgave her for destroying my penny collection.

This major psychic injury might have predisposed my neuronal pathways for the emotions of rage, agitation, confusion and, possibly, depression.

(4) Failure in Adolescent Love

When I was seventeen and in my final year of my blue-collar high school, my uncle offered me a job in his new service station, which was being built in an affluent neighborhood. I leapt at the opportunity.

One summer day, a girl my age drove in for service and I was smitten. Yet, it took me almost four weeks to build up enough courage to ask her out. When I did, she quickly accepted. What followed was an awkward but educationally rewarding "romance" in which I learned that my family was poor. I remember feeling bewilderment that her home was carpeted. I had never seen such a thing. Many other things amazed me. She had her own large bedroom while I shared a tiny one with my brother. She had three closets full of clothes, while I had five shirts and a few pairs of jeans. Her parents belonged to a country club. I didn't know what one was. Her father was a lawyer for a big downtown company, while mine made oil-field tools with his hands. Both of her parents were graduates of colleges. I didn't know what colleges were. Her Christmases were abundant, while mine were meager. But despite our material and social differences that made me feel quite inferior, and despite the stress I constantly felt when I was with her, I declared myself to be in love. We became a couple and started going to movies and Young Methodist Fellowship. I took dance lessons, rented tuxedos and took her to dances at her country club, which her mother paid for. I watched others and learned how to use napkins and utensils. I learned how to greet people, to shake hands firmly, to use wit in conversations and to praise the dresses and beauty of my sweetheart's friends. I learned about colleges and ended up going to one. I was a year ahead of her, so in my freshman year at Texas A&M, she was a senior in high school.

At college, I was miserable. I worried constantly that I was "losing" her. Still, I made two really good friends, one from New York and one from California, both, like my sweetheart, well above me in social class. My sweetheart encouraged me to invite my new friends to spend a long weekend in my home. I was overjoyed and set up the weekend with my mother.

When, however, I drove my friends into the driveway of my humble home, my delusions quickly evaporated. Not only were my friends mortified with cultural shock, so was my family. My two friends were bewildered by a home with linoleum on every floor, tiny rooms, sagging wall-paper moist with humidity, an attic fan that whirred loudly, beds with unmatched 'linens' and, at meals, plastic place sittings of whimsical beauty.

I was blindsided by everyone's embarrassment, especially that of my mother who had encouraged the weekend. It was, and still is, the most awkward experience of my life.

Quickly, I took my friends to my sweetheart's home, hoping to undo my embarrassment. But no, that too was to be a time of crushing reality, not of delusion. I watched with disbelieving eyes as my sweetheart and my friend from New York combined like hydrogen and oxygen. Their faces gleamed, their eyes danced, their voices fell into rhythm, they danced the Charleston to records, they sang together as the other friend played the piano, they compared their genealogies, talked about New York City and praised the breed of each other's dog. To nail home my feeling of total failure, my sweetheart's mother brought out refreshments for everyone except me.

This event of indescribable humiliation caused my first severe depression. In that condition, I failed out of Texas A&M.

This major adolescent psychic event might have predisposed my neuronal pathways for the emotions of restlessness, agitation, sleeplessness, racing thoughts, lethargy, apathy, difficulties in thinking, confusion and depression.

Step Three: Kindling

(a) My Adult Stresses Immediately Proceeding Kindling

I completed my college education at the University of Houston. Upon graduation in 1961, I "escaped" my family by joining the Navy (without knowledge at the time that I was repeating Daddy Ray's pattern). I eventually became, because of my color-blindness, a supply officer assigned to the U.S.S. Boston, home-ported in Boston. There I met and married a woman far higher on the social scale than my high school sweetheart. She was the daughter of an affluent family and had graduated from one of the East's "Seven Sisters" colleges.

Intelligent and well educated, my wife quickly learned to program an early computer at MIT, where she worked as a research assistant for a professor. Less intelligent and less well educated, I earned less money than she did in the early years of our marriage.

Cultural differences arose almost immediately. My wife would not wear the presents that I bought for her on my Navy cruises, presents that my mother and sisters would have considered exotic and beautiful. To please her, I applied to the Harvard and MIT Business Schools, knowing that I wasn't qualified. Nevertheless, I felt great shame when the letters of rejection arrived. To please her, I went along with her desires for big, beautiful houses in nice neighborhoods, then poorly endured the financial binds required, probably because they recreated the financial insecurities of my childhood.

We differed decisively, sometimes bitterly over how to rear our children. Having been reared that way, my wife favored autocratic methods; having been reared that way, I favored democratic methods.

Having been "to the Manor born", my wife craved to live in the East and to have little to do with my family. I also wanted to live away from my family, but I wanted to live away from hers, too. That tension, plus my ambition to make something of myself led to business promotions that resulted in three moves, to New Jersey, California and Illinois, not one of which my wife approved.

Despite these differences, both of us adored our children and organized our lives around them, keeping our arguments and differences "behind closed doors". The move to California, however, stressed the marriage to the breaking point. When we moved there, she would not help me purchase our new home. I bought a home that we could afford (in Palo Alto, now in the heart of "Silicon Valley"). My wife hated it.

Still, for the first time, not just in my marriage but in my life as well, I was truly happy. Something of an intellectual, I worked for an educational publisher developing and selling textbooks. My wife, however, was truly miserable. Knowing that she had been in on the beginning of the computer revolution and had given it up to rear children full time made her life as a mom bittersweet. I also traveled a lot, which deprived her of parenting help and adult companionship. Of major importance, her family didn't approve of California, and she felt isolated and lonely.

Without question, my greatest contribution to our marriage stresses came from the early childhood training of my neuronal pathways. I had been trained for the emotions of anxiety (fear), rage, restlessness, agitation and racing thoughts, sometimes combined with lethargy, apathy, difficulties in thinking, outright confusion and depression. Such emotions were not present at all times, especially in the early years of our marriage. Nor were my occasional feelings of ecstasy. I, of course, never once thought my emotions unusual. I assumed that everyone was like me. To a degree they were. But unknown to me at the time, my pre-dispositions, when put under enough stress, would cross me over the imaginary line called "normal" and into the wilderness called "psychotic".

By age thirty-five, when I was a two to three martini drinker at night, I began to experience recurring depression. I did not understand its source, but I intuitively guessed that it came from alcohol. I began to fear that I had inherited my father's alcoholism. One Christmas Eve, while decorating our tree with my wife and children, and listening to John Denver sing, "Please, Daddy, Don't Get Drunk This Christmas", I poured my martini down the drain and stopped drinking hard liquor forever. It took me another five years to stop drinking beer and wine, but I eventually did. I have been alcohol free since age forty-one. But while drinking alcohol triggered depressions, becoming alcohol free has not eliminated my depressions. Clearly, my depression has many mothers.

After ten years in Palo Alto, and ten years of increasing tension between us, I redeemed my promise that, if she were unhappy in California, I would move my wife back to the East. I resigned from the publishing company and took a job in Chicago, intending to complete the move east at a later opportunity.

But the further I drove from California the more deeply depressed I became. I truly loved Palo Alto and hated to leave it. In the Chicago area, we had bought another big beautiful house in a rich neighborhood and I knew what was coming. We could barely afford it, even on my new, larger salary. We couldn't keep our children dressed like their peers. An executive in my new company, I didn't have money to go to lunch with my colleagues. Before working the first month in my new job, I was already trying to figure out how to increase my income.

Once again our pushme-pullyou relationship had achieved a sort of stasis, only this time she was very happy and I was miserable. The lack of sunlight in winter greatly affected my continuing depressions for the worse. My boys were both learning disabled and gifted, and the oldest had a right-left dominance problem. They performed poorly in school and in all sports except soccer, in which they excelled. Determined to keep the self-esteem of my sons high, I started an age-group soccer program, which my wife opposed. She had just given birth to our third child and wanted my time devoted to her and our baby daughter.

I tried to do both, but I did not give up soccer, a decision that generated a great deal of stress. I felt that I had a father's obligation to all of my children, not just to the newest. I didn't feel that I could abandon my boys as strangers in a new community. I had ripped them out of their old support group and felt responsible for helping them establish a new one. So I persevered, and my soccer program became a roaring success. But it required tremendous effort on my part. I put more hours into soccer than into my day job or my role of helpmate.

Meanwhile, my new job quickly became another source of tremendous stress. I had been hired by an Executive Vice President to modernize the marketing of a division. But modernization was the last thing the division's president wanted. I became, in effect, a pawn between the Executive Vice President and the Division President. In stalemate and growing confusion, both at home and at work, I could not achieve what I had promised to the Executive Vice President. It was the first time that I had failed since becoming an adult. My anxieties soared.

At some point in this extremely high stress period at home and work, my wife asked me to add a male neighbor (married with children) to my soccer board, which met weekly. I did so, delighted to have a new helper.

With one success, soccer, and two never relenting stresses, my marriage and my job, I slipped into a deep depression in which I lost pleasure in everything except my children. In that condition (in 1981), I stumbled into a new, high-paying job in Philadelphia. I thought I had solved two problems, that of improving my financial condition by replacing a horrible job with a high-paying very promising one, and that of fulfilling my promise to my wife to move her back east. When my new Boss called to tell me that the job was mine, I thought my problems were solved. Significantly, however, my depression did not lift.

(b) My Kindling Eruption

Between jobs, my family and I, and the neighbor who my wife not only wanted on the soccer board, but also wanted on our vacation (with one of his children, but without his wife), went backpacking in Wyoming's Wind River Mountains. In my preoccupation, or innocence, or stupidity, or depression, I never picked up on the reason for my neighbor's presence. The moment that I finally figured it out was my moment of kindling.

My wife and I were cleaning up supper in an 11,000-foot camp. My wife suddenly decided that we needed more water. I thought it odd. The dishes were almost done and we still had plenty of water. But off she went in the last of the evening light, carrying our fabric water carrier and a flashlight to the nearby stream. From the tent, our two-year-old began to cry. I went to the tent to comfort my daughter, and from there watched my wife and neighbor through the netting of the zippered door. I was astounded to realize that it wasn't water that my wife sought, but the companionship of our neighbor. In a fog of disbelief I watched their every move, their brushes against each other, their holding hands, their long stares into each other's eyes.

At that moment, I felt as if my brain were on fire. It was as if something hot began to spread from the inside out. I moaned and held my head as if it were going to burst. I rubbed my forehead against the floor of the tent, tears storming from my eyes. My universe became completely disordered. I couldn't stop crying and I couldn't stop the pain in my head. Not wanting my children to hear me in such a pathetic condition, and feeling immensely slow, as if wading through cold molasses, I left and walked to the shore of the lake. By sunup, I was still there, not having slept the entire night. The part of my mind that dealt with normal things was gone. I could not recall the name of my new boss, nor of my old one. I could not remember what day it was. I could not remember how to cook pancakes for my boys. I had no appetite. I couldn't stop crying. My confusion was the scariest thing that I had ever experienced. I truly thought that I had lost my mind.

At that point, my wife informed me that she would not be moving to Philadelphia. She was in love with the neighbor. She would stay in Chicago and marry him. My identity and self-esteem, which were anchored in my family, were smashed.

- Note how similar my loss of adult love is to my loss of adolescent love. In both, I lost love objects to friends, in the earlier one to a friend from a social order similar to that of my high school sweetheart, in the latter to a friend from an intellectual order similar to that of my wife's (he was a computer specialist). It is possible, according to my research, that I experienced both sets of emotions, those of my adult loss and those of my adolescent loss, at the same moment.

Step Four: Intermittent Reinforcements

"When the sun is in the seventh house, and Jupiter aligns with Mars…." So goes the lyric from *This is the Age of Aquarius*, one of the many fabulous songs from the musical *Hair*. I think often of that lyric because that is the way I perceive that I kindled into BPII. First and most importantly, I probably had the genetic inheritance, perhaps from both sides of my family. Secondly, I had early childhood stresses. Everyone, of course, has early childhood stresses, some far worse than mine. Everyone also has adult stresses, some far worse than mine. But most people have healthy amygdalas that keep the memories of their stresses separate while I probable don't. More than likely, I kindled into a BPII event because my amygdala confused my childhood stresses with my adult stresses. And when those two sets of stresses were aligned like Jupiter and Mars, I became a candidate for permanent BPII.

But just a candidate. To graduate from a kindling event into permanent BPII requires more alignments. The kindling event must be reinforced with similar stresses in a random way. By "random" I mean unpredictable in occurrence, severity and duration. In other words, Jupiter must align with Mars often, but not regularly.

My reinforcing events occurred while attempting to save my marriage.

I had no option but to leave my wife and children in Chicago while I went to my new job in Philadelphia. I could not return to my Chicago job, and there was a mortgage to satisfy and children to clothe and feed.

Once in Philadelphia, I was unable to concentrate on business. The trauma of my wife's transformation, and fear over what was happening behind my back in Chicago, occupied my mind to the exclusion of normal duties and pleasures.

During this period, I began to hallucinate that my life was unreal. In that state, I performed my new job poorly. My new boss was not pleased. My anxieties soared.

I became confused by new hallucinations. I felt that my skin was melting from my bones. I felt that people in the office and on the streets were staring at me, and were disgusted that my skin was dripping so. Shamed senseless, however, I would not talk to anyone about my problems.

I could afford to fly home every other weekend. There and on the telephone, I tried desperately and fruitlessly to save my marriage. Coldly, my wife kept repeating that she loved my neighbor very much and planned to marry him. Furthermore, she would not agree to sell the Chicago house (that we owned jointly) and move to Philadelphia.

I developed volcanic anger over my wife and my neighbor. Unable to sleep either in Philadelphia or in Chicago, I began walking the streets at night. Yet, to protect my children's feelings, I never discussed their mother's behavior with them. Nor, for the same reason, did I discuss it with any of my many friends in the community.

One Sunday night, following a weekend in Chicago empty of accomplishment, I began crying on the plane and was unable to stop. By Monday morning, still crying, I finally realized that I needed professional help. My mother-in-law, a wonderful woman, helped me find a psychiatrist and I arranged to see him daily after work.

The psychiatrist treated me, correctly at the time, with the antidepressant *Elavil*. It is now known that the family of tricyclic antidepressants, of which *Elavil* is one, triggers mania in people with genetic weaknesses in that direction. My taking *Elavil* was a seminal event. Already kindled and endlessly bombarded with intermittent psychological blows, I moved into a mixed state of depression and dysphoric (sad) mania.

Intermittent reinforcements never relented. About six months after my arrival at the new job, displeased with my job performance and probably not blind to my confused affect, my new boss made me talk about what was going on. I was unable to do so without crying. I expected to be fired soon after the conversation. But to my astonished surprise, my boss offered to buy our Chicago house. In elation and denial, I called my wife with the good news. It wasn't good news to her. She rejected the offer out of hand. My boss, when told, ceased being understanding. Anxiety over my likely loss of income soared. Over and over I ruminated, "How could I ever support my family when I had lost my mind". At times I worried that we would all die.

My wife finally agreed to visit me in Philadelphia. I was elated. At last, the dam had burst. I planned to show her a house that I had found, the kind she liked, a real beauty in a very nice township. But she had no desire to see the house or any of the neighborhoods. In deep depression and frazzled from anxiety, rage, depression, agitation, sleeplessness, and racing thoughts, I realized that she was just going through the motions of a visit, probably to satisfy her mother. Even then, however, I could not break out of my denial that our marriage was over.

Eleven months after my arrival in Philadelphia, it was apparent that I was about to be fired. It was over. I was going to loose everything. Then, in the strangest pushme-pullyou of the entire drama, my wife decided that she wasn't in love with my neighbor after all. Now she wanted to move to Philadelphia very much. My hallucination that life was unreal was confirmed.

The axe fell within days of her call. For the first time in my life, at age forty-two, I was fired. Now I considered myself to be a "double failure", both in marriage and in business. Worst, my mind was dominated by uncontrollable emotions that interfered with even my slightest efforts to concentrate. Even so, something more horrible was yet to come. My Philadelphia psychiatrist, acting in good faith upon the feedback that I provided him after having read "Mood Swings" by Fevie, and the advice of a research psychiatrist at the University of Pennsylvania, arranged for me to begin lithium therapy when I returned to Chicago.

Step Five: The Illness Becomes Automatic

It is now known that *lithium carbonate* is an effective mood stabilizer for roughly 50% of manic-depressives. [60] I belong to the other 50% that do not respond to *lithium carbonate*. The drug did slow down my quick thinking and it eliminated my sex drive altogether, the absence of which profoundly affected my ability to rebuild my marriage. It also made my

---

60   Post, R.M.; Ketter, T.A.; Pazzaglia, P.J.; Denicoff, K.; George, M. S.; Callahan, A.; Leverich, G.; Fry, M., (1996). Rational polypharmacy in the bipolar affective disorders. *Epilepsy-Res-Suppl., 11*: 153-80.

hands tremble noticeably, which made me feel old and feeble. But it did not stabilize my moods nor relieve my feelings that everything was coming apart, including my mind.

Chicago

My return to my home in Chicago was humiliating. I had left it a year previously admired for founding the town's age group soccer program. Now I was back without a job and receiving unemployment insurance for the first time in my life. I was certain that everyone was gossiping behind my back about my strange doings. Yet I would not talk to my friends about what had really gone on for fear of embarrassing my wife, my children and myself.

My wife very much needed understanding and forgiveness. I, however, was just too ill to give it. I had lost the job that would have allowed her to live as she desired, as well as to send our children to college. Now I was fired and forty-four, an age when it is very hard to find good jobs. We would be lucky to keep our home. In my frustration and humiliation, and feeling like a dead man on *lithium carbonate*, I was unable to meet her needs. I was confused, sometimes dizzy, lethargic and apathetic in the extreme and had considerable difficulties in thinking.

By this time, my illness was either automatic or well on its way to becoming such. I continued to hallucinate that my skin was melting from my bones. I developed a pronounced "startle reaction" for sounds large and small, telephone rings, my wife speaking, my children's shouts, doors banging. My reaction to each startle was a pounding heart, a throbbing head and anger. I moved my job search efforts into the basement of our home.

In 1983, Chicago and the rest of the "rust belt" were in recession. I received very few job interviews. When I did, I interviewed like a slow, shaky old man. I received no job offers for almost a year. It seemed impossible to me, but the evidence was incontrovertible, I had become undesirable as a spouse and as a business manager simultaneously. A truly dreadful feeling quickly followed. I became guilt ridden that I was a bad father, that I had passed on "bad genes" and that my "strange behaviors" were bad examples to my children. And worst of all, it was becoming increasingly evident that I would not be able to pay for my children's college education. In my ever-churning confusion, I felt like a three-time failure. My depression seemed unendurable.

At last, a large Chicago company offered me a job in Denver at four-fifths of the pay of the Philadelphia job. I surged out of depression into a happy, optimistic mania. Once again, everything was "solved". The expensive Chicago house would be replaced with a less costly one and we would be able to educate our children. I would go off *lithium carbonate* and get my sex urge back. My wife and I would be able to truly reconcile. We would be able to play in the Rocky Mountains whenever we pleased.

But my wife quickly and firmly said that she was not going to move to Denver. She had already moved three times in their marriage. That was enough for her. Chicago was a big place. It was unreasonable for me to assume that I could not find a job there.

I, however, was in mania and feeling omnipotent. Exercising the poor judgment for which manic-depressives are famous[61], I accepted the job anyway. Off I went to Denver, feeling considerable (and false) *noblesse oblige* to make the hard decisions for my family. Along the way, I threw away my *lithium carbonate*. I needed all of my mental energy, now. I could no long afford to waste it on a drug that made me feel horrible.

Denver

Soon after my arrival at my new job, a deputy sheriff served me with divorce papers. I erupted with fury and crashed into depression. I could

---

61   Ghaemi, A.N.; Stoll, A.L.; Pope, H.G. (1995). Lack of insight in bipolar disorder. *The Journal of Nervous and Mental Disease, 183,* 7: 464-467

no longer deny my feelings of betrayal. Of all my bad judgements, perhaps the worse was putting myself in a location where I had no support group. My children and friends were in Chicago. My birth family was in Texas. I had no shoulder to lean on, no wise counselor.

Divorce proceedings lasted about eight months. Each court motion and telephone call from my wife and my lawyer doubled and redoubled my anger and depression. Once again, my reaction to my wife's behavior was causing me to perform a job poorly. Yet, I could not bring myself to fight her. The grounds of her divorce petition were "mental cruelty". Before a judge, she would claim my many suspected, and mostly imaginary, affairs; I would counter with her behavior with the neighbor in Chicago. It would be messy, sensational and no good for the children. I proposed a settlement and she accepted one very favorable to her.

By now, my BPII was automatic. I alternated between high, optimistic energy and low, deeply depressed energy. Things mental kept coming apart. I became inconsistent in almost every thing I did. By the end of my year's trial time, I failed to meet my business plan goals and was fired from the Denver job.

With more bad judgement, I used money from the divorce settlement to start a business in Denver. I failed at that, too.

Ft. Worth

I moved to Texas to be near my sisters. Once again, I tried to start a business only to fail. I began to take sales jobs, but because of anger and inconsistent performance, I could not hold them for longer than four months. When I could no longer pay child support, suicide ideations began. Eventually, I packed up my valuables and shipped them to my children. Then I drove to the mountains above Denver to overdose on *Elavil*. I was, however, unable to write a goodbye letter to my daughter. From Boulder, I called an uncle in Houston. The uncle wired me money, and I went there for my first stay in a psychiatric ward.

Houston

I arrived at the Houston Veteran's Administration Hospital depressed and withdrawn. I received personal therapy from a doctor whom I greatly admired and daily group therapy with vets suffering a rainbow of psychological problems. Once again, I was put on *lithium carbonate*, the only drug approved for BPII in 1987. The doctor whom I admired was a Freudian. Her skills in group therapy and insights in individual therapy dazzled me. With the fresh vision that comes from a suicide attempt, I soaked up her knowledge. For the first time, I confronted the idea that my adult mental problems might be the fruit of my reactions to my childhood problems.

When my six-week stay at the VA ended, I followed my Freudian doctor to the Baylor Medical School of Psychiatry, where she was to do a ninth year of internship. For more than a year, we met and worked very hard in two major areas of Freudian psychology: (1) how adulthood is spent attempting to work out the unresolved problems of childhood, and (2) the secrets that we keep from ourselves, called "denial" by Freud.

For most of the year I was on *lithium carbonate*, which slowed down but did nothing to stop my depression. My Freudian doctor taught me a process for relieving my depressions. First, I would identify what had made me recently angry. Then I would search my childhood memories for anger events similar to current ones (a painful process), substituting current symbols for original ones, ex-wife for Mother, myself for Father, my children for myself. Once the associations over time were made, and the time confusion and the symbol confusion were understood, the anger and depression abated.

Totally impressed with what I called my "Freudian depression licker", I went off *lithium carbonate* again. Soon thereafter, my trusted doctor accepted a position out of the city. Alone with my demons once more, I attempted to keep my depression in check using her methods. I never cared about keeping mania in check, of course. Who would? Mania is always fun. For me it is a period of high energy and heightened pleasures. Eventually I would learn that to breakeven with BPII, that I would have to give up mania. But before I learned that, mania was my reward for enduring depression.

Using her Freudian method, I was partially successful in modifying depression. The process worked temporarily, not permanently. Freud, of course, conceived of depression as a mind problem, a neurotic reaction to a life situation. And, indeed, such a process does cause some depression. But it is now known that some depression is caused by faulty brain chemistry, and that is the kind from which I suffer. Unmedicated and uncounseled, therefore, my depressions (and occasional mania) kept coming in endless waves of misery and ecstasy.

I believe that my trusted doctor's Freudian methods failed because, in accordance with the Post Model of Affective Illness, my illness had by that time become automatic. In the beginning, huge stresses of betrayal and loss of income kindled my illness. Three years of intermittent stresses followed, the most significant of which were failure to heal my marriage, failure to earn money for my family and an unwanted divorce. By the time that I met my Freudian doctor, my illness had graduated into accelerated episodes with the episodes themselves as the stimulant.

Step Six: Containment is Achieved With Drugs

Once again, I was unable to maintain employment. I went through too many jobs to count, mostly contract sales jobs. I tried to sell cable subscriptions door to door, medical insurance, beds, siding, credit cards, cookbooks, electricity audits and a host of other things, all unsuccessfully. By August of 1994, fourteen years after my kindling and as tired as death of my relentless waves of depression, I entered my suicide cycle. I packed my car with valuables for my children and set off to complete the task, "properly" this time.

I left my car and valuables for my children, then went into a wilderness and overdosed on *Elavil*. I hallucinated, but did not die. My sons retrieved me and took me to a local VA Hospital. There I was put on *Trilafon*, a neuroleptic, and, once again, *lithium carbonate.*

Upon release from the hospital, I lived temporarily with a son and attempted to find work near my children. I failed. Once again I attempted suicide. I failed. My son, acting with "tough love", evicted me.

At this point in the evolution of my illness' personality, I was not only rapid-cycling between depression and mania I was also rapid-cycling in suicide attempts. In a state of sleepless agitation and soaring anxiety, I called a cousin near Shreveport, Louisiana. He agreed to take me in. A true Christian, he shared everything he owned with me until I regained my sanity.

At my first appointment in the Shreveport VA Mental Health Clinic, I was discovered to have *Tardive Dyskinesia*, a palsy illness induced in some recipients of neuroleptic drugs like *Trilafon*. My *Trilafon* prescription was discontinued. *Zoloft*, an antidepressant in the *Prozac* family was added to my course of *lithium carbonate*. That drug combination didn't work either. Soon thereafter, I attempted suicide for a fourth time. I failed. I entered the psychiatric ward of the Shreveport VA Hospital in December 1994, complaining that *Zoloft* made me feel like a fetus.

My prescription was changed from *Zoloft* to *Paxil*, and the black dog of depression slowly let me go. Its effect was not immediate. It took time for the drug to get into each of my brain's 10 billion neurons and it took more time to discover the appropriate level of dosage. I began at 20 mg, went up as high as 50 mg, then settled at 40 mg before I felt that my depression was finally under control. The other shoe dropped in October of 1995 when *valproic acid* became available. Within weeks of starting *valproic acid*, peace returned to my mind like a gentle dew from heaven. That was a very emotional time for me. For the first time in fourteen years, I felt that I had not lost my mind. It would be another five years before I would call myself "optimistic". But the corner had been turned.

But though I thought that I was ready for society, society wasn't ready for me.

Step Seven: The Continued Evolution of the Illness

(a) Psychopharmacology, 1981 to 2000

Year	Mood Stabilizer	Neuroleptic	Antidepressant	Results
1981			Elavil, 20 mg	Triggered mania
1982	Lithium, 1,000 mg			Slowed mania; ineffective for depression
1983-87	On and off lithium			Slowed mania, no depression relief, one suicide attempt
1987-94	Freudian methods, no drugs			Increased mania and depression, one suicide attempt
1994		Trilafon, 8 mg		Speech less tangential; thoughts continued to race
1994	Lithium, 300 mg	Trilafon, 8 mg		Slowed racing thoughts, one suicide attempt, tardive dyskinesia
1995	Lithium, 300 mg		Zoloft, 50 mg	One suicide attempt
	Lithium, 300 mg		Paxil, 20 mg	Less frequent and severe depression

Lithium, 900 mg	Paxil, 30 mg	One vital depression
Lithium, 900 mg	Paxil, 50 mg	Headaches, sleepy, very lethargic
Lithium, 900 mg	Paxil, 40 mg	Depressions ended, mania continued
10/ 1995 Valproic Acid, 2000 mg	Paxil, 40 mg	Amazing peace
1/ 2000 Valproic Acid, 2000 mg	Paxil 40 mg	Outbreaks of anger, agitation,confusion.
2/ 2000 Valproic Acid, 2000 mg	Prozac 20 mg	Crying jags, very tired
3/ 2000 Valproic Acid, 2000 mg	Paxil 20 mg	Stability, optimism, high energy
6/ 2000 Valproic Acid, 2000 mg	Paxil 20 mg	Major mood swing, followed by anger blowup.

This chart presents my nineteen-year drug history from 1981, when I kindled into BPII, until the year 2000. Post's research indicates that my illness is organic; that is, that it will continue to evolve. Keeping stable, therefore, will probably require changes to my drugs as my illness grows into new regions of my brain.[62] Note especially that Post recommends adding new drugs to old drugs, not replacing old drugs with new ones. His research shows that evolution of the illness involves new neurons. Thus the original neurons involved in the original illness should continue to be treated with the drugs that were originally effective. Upon breakout from the original containment, the newly ill neurons should

---

62   Post, R.M. & Weiss, S. B., (1995). F.E. Bloom (Ed.), & D.J. Kupfer (Ed.), *Psychopharmacology: The Forth Generation of Progress.* (p 1162, "Tolerance Emergence During Long Term Prophylaxis"). Raven Press,. Ltd., New York. **See Book**

be treated with new drugs effective for the new breakout. Discovering the right drug for a breakout will require new rounds of trial and error testing.

Note that such a breakout may have begun in my illness. I was mostly stable from October of 1995 until August of 1999. Then, as revealed by the following sequence, things began to become less stable:

Date	Reaction
8/99	Severe two week depression
9/99	Recurring outbursts of irrational anger
10/99	One day of migraine aura in eyes, one major dizzy spell
11/99	Beginning of usual holiday depression
12/99	Worst holiday depression since going on *valproic acid*
1/00	Very sleepy, irritable for almost the entire month
2/00	Loss of most pleasures. Aggressive, angry behavior in my Psychotherapy Group. Antidepressant changed from 40 mg Paxil to 20 mg Prozac [an error according to Post].
3/00	Major confusion, three major crying jags, slow and sleepy. Antidepressant changed from 20 mg Prozac to 20 mg Paxil
4/00	Almost immediate relief from confused, depressed feelings, followed by two months of very stable feelings
5/00	On May 28, outbursts of irrational anger over my uncle, brother and dog
6/00	From June 4 to June 9, a sharp depression followed by hypomania that lasted until June 15th. Beginning June 22, a sharp decline into depression, anger and sleep disturbance.

Michael Crawford

(b) A Summary of Social Functioning

As mentioned earlier, Carl Menninger conceived of mental illness as a continuum of social incompatibility, a concept that resonates strongly with my experiences. Schizophrenics, for example, are almost totally withdrawn from society. Psychotics mostly are. The depressed sometimes are. Those with behavior problems do not withdraw, but participate poorly.

My stages of social incompatibility may be summarized as follows:

Year	Stage of Incompatibility
Prior to 1981	Highly functional in society prior to my kindling event.
1981	Still functional, but fighting the urge to withdraw
1982 to 1995	My period of ineffective medication and on-again, off-again counseling, the time when my illness became automatic, when I withdrew from society, climaxed, in 1994, by my suicide cycle.
1995	Effective drugs and counseling at last.
1996 to 1998	An extremely awkward time when, with encouragement and support from by my counselor but very little confidence in myself, and with repeated false starts, I attempted to reenter society. I failed.
1999 to 2000	Small, successful, confidence-boosting steps in reentering society. This time, I am succeeding.

Today I am somewhat reintegrated into society. I belong to a church that has helped me in immeasurable ways, although I continue to struggle with feelings that I don't fit in. With full knowledge of my background, my local School District allows me to substitute-teach. The Social Security Administration supports me with disability income. Though I continue to live alone, I have tried twice to establish relationships with members of the fair sex. Both failed because of me, not them. I continue to feel that I am flawed. Having experienced a lot of it, I expect prejudice. I feel claustrophobic in crowds. I require a lot of individual quiet time.

My future? I will always be affectively ill. Drugs will contain my illness, but not cure it. My continuing task will be to continue building a new mind around my old one that will allow me to correct the faulty thoughts and feelings from my ever-present past. It will be a never-ending process. But I can do that.

6

How to Breakeven
with Bipolar Illness

It is estimated that the prevalence of unipolar illness is 21.3% for women and 12.7% for men. The prevalence of bipolar illness is estimated to be 1.6% with equal gender distribution. Forty percent of bipolar patients are inadequately treated or not treated at all. Twenty-five percent of bipolars attempt suicide, and 11% to 19% of them succeed. Relapse rates are over 90% and are often accompanied by significant disruptions to social, educational and occupational roles. Those afflicted have to struggle, often with their own loved ones and sometimes with unread professionals, with misconceptions and myths about their illness–that it can be willed away; that it gets better with time; that is not severe; that rapid response to treatment is the norm; that medications should be discontinued when the acute episode has passed; and that medications can be stopped and restarted.[63]

No bipolar will ever be "cured". Well periods can last for years, but true bipolar always returns. Breakeven with the illness is possible, however. It's just a matter of learning to live with it. Because every case of BPII is different, there is no "One Size Fits All" breakeven roadmap.

---

63   Leverich, G.S. & Post, R.M., (1998). Life charting of affective disorders. *The International Journal of Neuropsychiatric Medicine, 3 (5)*: 21-37

Each of us must create our own. What follows worked for me; maybe it will help you, maybe it won't. My sincere hope is that it will, at least, get you started.

In a Nutshell

In a nutshell, the way I have approached breakeven is to try to make it visible to my mind's eye: to reverse, as it were, the frost of mental illness and resume the experimental action called "thinking". Remember always that you are mentally ill, not mentally retarded.

This, of course, is far easier said than done because our brains are universes unto themselves. You may be properly or improperly medicated. Your stresses may be unabating. Additionally, your kindling event may not be as depersonalizing as mine or may be more depersonalizing than mine.

Depersonalization is a good place to start. Here is its definition from the ©Online Medical Dictionary:

> An alteration in the perception of the self so that the usual sense of one's own reality is lost, manifested in a sense of unreality or self-estrangement, in changes of body image, or in a feeling that one does not control his own actions and speech.

Under such circumstances, even if unmedicated or improperly medicated, it is still possible to approach visibility, to see BPII at work "through a glass darkly".

Recognizing the Illness

The Invisible Part

BPII probably begins with a genetic inheritance of a faulty limbic systems, that part of the brain that is suspected of being the repository of feelings and the operating system of memory. You might also, as a child, been the recipient of BPI-type behavior in which you might have been environmentally "taught" by your parents how to turn your mental stress into depression or mania.

If you are the inheritor of a faulty limbic system, then you are a candidate for BPI. Not all candidates, however, develop the illness. In metaphor, genetics is the vine upon which the illness grows and the vine may very well be present in you; but the fruit of the vine is produced only when there is nutritious soil (certain childhood stresses) and sunlight (certain adulthood stresses). Every childhood has stress, of course. But it isn't the stress that's the precursor to BPI, it is a child's **response** to the stress that is. For example, one child might "train" its neuronal pathways to "do something mental" with its stresses and another might train its neuronal pathways to "do something physical" with it, such as grinding teeth.

Most childhood stress can be reduced to a single word: fear. In childhood, mental discharge of the stress of fear might include the behaviors of extreme shyness, hyperactivity, nightmares, etc. Such discharges are repeated in direct relationship to the incidence of fear experienced in childhood. Repeated fear yields repeated "training" of neuronal pathways, which eventually yields later pathological behaviors. Overall, a little more that 1-% of the population in both sexes, all races, and all parts of the world develop bipolar disorder.[64]

Only brains with childhood buds of pathological behavior are candidates for bipolar disorder. Even so, an emotionally shattering (kindling) event is required to ignite the illness. If such an event never happens, bipolar disorder probably never develops.

---

64 Rush, J.A., M.D. & Suppes, T., M.D., (1998) "What are the new treatments for bipolar disorder?", *The Harvard Mental Health Letter*, January, 74 Fenwood Road, Boston, MA 02115

A kindling event only kindles a small fire, perhaps a single episode of depression or mania. For bipolar disorder to fully flower, intermittent reinforcement is required. That is, additional emotionally shattering events must occur in an irregular sequence (which is the way most lives unfold). Your incredible brain remembers each emotionally shattering event and responds with depression and/or mania events.

Just as it learned and remembered responses to childhood fear, your brain learns and remembers mania and depression responses to adulthood fear. After a certain number of irregular reinforcements to your adult fears, it no longer needs shattering emotional events to stimulate its bipolar responses. Rather, it uses its fabulous memory to recall mania and depression events whenever current emotional events remotely resemble emotional events remembered from the past. Post calls this the stage of "episodes begatting episodes".

The Visible Part

The visible part of bipolar begins after kindling and reinforcement. In the beginning, however, even though this behavior will be perfectly visible to your physician and loved ones, it will be invisible to you. In fact, you will never be able to "see" your bipolar behavior until you are stable on drugs and have begun to compare yourself to other bipolars in group therapy. A list of the most obviously visible bipolar behavior would include:

- You are overwhelmed with grief.
- You can't stop crying.
- You confuse hours of the day, days of the weeks, even months of the year. You miss appointments and deadlines and can't remember the names of bosses and fellow workers.
- You stop taking care of your appearance. You might even stop taking showers.

- Even at work, you can't wake up.
- You lose all sense of pleasure, even in sex.
- You get fired.
- You get fired from another job, then another, and another and another and another.
- You secretly spend money on get rich quick schemes and lose it all.
- For "no reason at all" your anger explodes.
- You begin to hallucinate.
- You begin to consider suicide.
- You begin to plan your suicide.
- You have inexplicable days when your optimism suddenly returns.
- You have inexplicable days when your energy suddenly returns.
- Your sex drive returns, perhaps is undeniable.
- You can't stop talking.
- You get a fabulous new job.
- Everyone loves you.
- You labor in vain to regain a lost love.
- You spend money freely, even money that you haven't yet earned.
- Your anger explodes "for no reason at all".
- You become overwhelmed by feelings of grief.
- You can't stop crying.
- And so on, *ad infinitum.*

The Essential Behaviors Following Recognition

The essential behaviors following recognition are:

- To go off all drugs, including alcohol.

- To put yourself under the care of a psychiatrist immediately; not a *psychologist*, who is trained to counsel, but who cannot prescribe medicine, but a *psychiatrist*, a medical doctor who can both counsel and prescribe medicine.

- To take the drugs that he or she prescribes precisely the way you are told. **DON'T EXPERIMENT WITH YOUR NEW DRUGS.** They will make you feel terrible in the beginning, perhaps for as long as five weeks. Furthermore, it may take a year or more to find the right dose. Remember, every case of bipolar disorder is different; thus, every person will react differently to each drug and/or combination of drugs. **DO NOT CURSE THE PROCESS.** Yes, it is trial and error. Accept it. Don't fight it. There is no other way. Cooperate with your physician and remember to give him or her precise feedback, preferably with a daily chart of your moods (see below).

- To openly discuss **all** thoughts of suicide with your most trusted confidant. When suicidal, always talk before taking action. Recognize that there are three steps in suicide: (1) thinking about it, (2) planning a method, (3) taking action, such as buying guns or drugs. Whenever you reach step (2), you **must** talk to a psychiatrist. Remember always that a mentally ill person has very poor judgement. What seems very logical to a deeply depressed person often seems humorously illogical when the mood changes.

- Finally, to find a support group and become a regular member (your psychiatrist will know of one). Group therapy is invaluable to breaking even with bipolar disorder. It is very unlikely that there is anything you have felt or experienced that someone else has not already been through. Even if yours is the worst case of bipolar disorder ever, the lessor cases will help make your own case visible.

A Mind Trick That Works

An illusion of the mind that has worked especially well for me is "I will become the playwright of my life." In this illusion, my life is a play and I have the choices of being the playwright, the director, an actor, or a member of the audience.

To use this mind trick, you must begin by recognizing yourself for what you (and all others) are in life, an actor. Place yourself in the audience and watch yourself on the stage (counselors and groups are invaluable in this step). If you don't like what you see, coach yourself like a director. If you really don't like what you see, rewrite the play like a playwright.

Attitudes That Improve Visibility and Recognition

Attitudes are important to visibility because what we say to ourselves is the most important conversation that we ever have, for the obvious reason that we trust ourselves more than anyone else. Therefore, we must be a good friend and a wise counselor to ourselves. The positive attitudes that you will need are important in total, not in sequence. Therefore, it is not possible to say, "start with this attitude, then move on to the next". Rather, you must apply positive attitudes upon your illness all at the same time. Here are the ones that worked for me.

"This mood will change."

When you are flying high in mania and overflowing with optimism, when you are exploring the depths of hell in depression and wishing for death, even if you are in a blessed well interval, you must say to yourself often, "this mood will change". When it does, you must not be surprised. Never say, "it's over", or "here I go again". Always say, "it's over temporarily", or "here I go again, but it won't last".

"I can do this."

I hated being told that I was "just a little bit psychotic". Here is how the "On Line Medical Dictionary" defines the word:

> A mental disorder characterized by gross impairment in reality testing as evidenced by delusions, hallucinations, markedly incoherent speech or disorganized and agitated behavior without apparent awareness on the part of the patient of the incomprehensibility of his behavior. The term is also used in a more general sense to refer to mental disorders in which mental functioning is sufficiently impaired as to interfere grossly with the patients capacity to meet the ordinary demands of life.
>
> Historically, the term has been applied to many conditions, for example manic depressive psychosis, that were first described in psychotic patients, although many patients with the disorder are not judged psychotic.

In my opinion of myself, I am in no way psychotic. Nor, in my opinion, have I ever been. Yet, doctors with eight years of training or more were telling me that I was. My reaction was immediate. I felt sorry for myself for quite awhile, imagined my life to be a Greek tragedy and grieved the loss of my family yet again. But eventually I was able to say, "O.K., I'm a little bit psychotic. That certainly explains why my marriage fell apart. Why I can't hold jobs, too. But that doesn't mean that I am a bad person. If I can find drugs that work for me, I won't be psychotic. I can do this."

"I will not give up."

If you experience the incomprehensibility of life turning upside down; if you are astounded that your loving wife is suddenly afraid of you; if you become paralyzed with anxiety over the fate of your children; if you are in terror because your doctor thinks you are mentally ill; if you lose your job, and your next job, and your next and your next and your next; if you realize that your drugs aren't magic bullets, and that they have unpleasant side effects; if you lose your sex drive, and the loss makes you feel less than human; if loneliness eats you up like a cancer; if you discover yourself about to commit suicide; if you find yourself in a psychiatric ward, then another, and another; the attitude that will pull you through is, "I will not give up".

"I will not get well until I admit that I'm sick."

Sweeping statements are almost always untrue, so I try very hard to avoid them. Yet, I can't think of a single case of bipolar disorder, including that of Dr. Kay Jamison, the much-published psychologist, the author of *An Unquiet Mind* and the co-author of a textbook on bipolar disorder, who did not go off their drugs for a period of time. Doing so seems to be part of learning about the illness. In my early years in bipolar disorder, a steady stream of doubt towards drugs and doctors ran constantly through my mind.

"Am I really as sick as the doctors think?"

"The drugs are worse than the illness."

"How do they expect me to lead a normal life when the drugs make me feel like a zombie?"

"I need to be a little manic to succeed at work."

Mania may well be the reason that we bipolars go off drugs. Mania is blissful. It acts upon the same region of the brain as does cocaine. In my experience, I was dependent upon it to make my way in the world. Giving it up meant giving up my uniqueness, my cutting edge, and my major strength. Indeed, if the illness were just mania, who would ever want to be "well" of it?

But the illness is not just mania. The piper of mania must be paid with the living death of depression, in my case, at a rough rate of four depressions for each one of mania. I hate to admit that it took me years to figure it out, but it did: to avoid depression, I must mania no more.

Then came the most difficult decision that I have ever had to make, in order to mania no more, I realized, required the admission that I was sick with an illness that I could not tackle alone. To "beat" the illness and return to something of a normal life, I would have to willingly give up my very precious previous identity, which was that of a "born to win" person, and place my future in the hands of psychiatrists and psychologists.

No sooner did I make the decision to do so, which turned out to be the smartest one I have ever made, than I began to be assailed by my family.

"You're not sick."

"You're letting doctors ruin you."

"Get off those drugs and back into church!"

And so on. But even stubbornness has a good side. I stuck with my decision because I knew something that no one else did, not even the doctors: What it is like to be whipsawed month after month after month by depression and mania. A life of drugs and doctors is glorious in comparison.

Many aphorisms appear unnatural when first considered.

"If you love your children, give them discipline."

"A teenager's greatest need is not to be needed."

"The child is the father of the man."

"Grief makes one hour two."

"One today is worth two tomorrows."

And so it is with, "Bipolars will not get well until they admit that they are sick." The admission is extraordinarily painful, and the psychic price is incalculable. But without it, I am convinced, bipolars will never breakeven with the illness.

"Without accurate communication from me, physicians are helpless."

Relationships with psychiatrists and psychologists remind me of a favorite *New Yorker* cartoon: A peacock, with its glorious tail spread to its maximum is looking down at a dusty sparrow and saying, "And now, let's talk of you".

One of your most important jobs as a bipolar disorder patient is to puff yourself up to peacock size and talk to your doctors as an equal. Why *must* you do this? Because each case of bipolar disorder is unique, that's why. Therefore, no amount of textbook learning, and no amount of "experience treating bipolar disorder" enables your doctors to treat you the way you uniquely feel unless you tell them precisely the way you uniquely feel.

Keeping a daily journal is highly recommended. Here is an entry from mine:

May 4, 1995 (while on 900 mg Lithium & 30 mg Paxil):

Outside my head: Home alone. Up at 5. Wrote well. O.K .day at work.

Inside my head: While waking up, heard female voices behind the bedroom walls.

Couldn't understand what they said.

Mood: Pessimistic, sleepy, headed down.

From your journal, you will be able to chart yourself by month. Here are the definitions needed to keep a chart:

The Continuum of Mania and Depression
As Defined In
The NIMH-LCM[65]

4.Severe Mania: much insistence by others that patient get medical attention, patient unable to function in any goal directed activity.

Symptoms: little or no sleep, delusional, invincible, explosive, hallucinatory, catatonic.

Functional Impairment: needs close supervision, has no judgement, puts self and others in danger, should be hospitalized.

3. High Moderate Mania: very significant difficulty with behavior and goal directed activities, can't focus, non-productive.

Symptoms: grandiose, very disruptive, little or no sleep, reckless, increases in energy and activities.

Functional Impairment: little or no judgement, not directable, outlandish behaviors, can't function at work.

2. Low Moderate Mania: noticeable impairment; others feedback about behavior; less productive, unfocused.

Symptoms: irritable/euphoric, intrusive, grandiose, increases in energy, decrease in sleep, increase in spending and phone calls.

Functional Impairment: poor judgement, sometimes disruptive at work and home, difficulty with goal-oriented activity.

---

65   Leverich, G.S. & Post, R.M., (1998). Life charting of affective disorders. *The International Journal of Neuropsychiatric Medicine, 3* (5): 21-37

1. Mild Mania: no impairment or mild impairment, functioning possibly enhanced.

    Symptoms: decrease in sleep, ebullient, energetic, more social, mildly pressured.

    Functional Impairment: little or no impairment can be focused and productive.

0. The Normal Range of Emotions

1. Mild Depression: no impairment to mild impairment.

    Symptoms: subjective distress, low mood, sleep and appetite O.K.

    Functional Impairment: functions well at work and at home, little or no impairment in social relationships.

2. Low Moderate Depression: noticeable impairment; some extra effort needed to function in usual social and occupational roles.

    Symptoms: decrease/increase in sleep and appetite, decreased energy and concentration, anxious, loss of normal pleasures, sucidal.

    Functional Impairment: some impairment at work and home, misses days from work, has to push self.

3. High Moderate Depression: very significant impairment; great effort needed to function in any role; barely scrapes by.

    Symptoms: retarded/agitated, very low energy, suicidal, withdrawn, poor hygiene, much difficulty reading or concentrating.

    Functional Impairment: great difficulty functioning, rarely goes to work, has to push self very hard.

4. Severe Depression: essentially incapacitated because of depression.

    Symptoms: immobilized, can't read or concentrate, mute or extremely agitated.

Functional Impairment: Isolated, or in bed, may be hospitalized.

Using the above definitions, create a Rhythm Chart for yourself such as this:

My Daily Rhythm Chart

Date: *June, 1995*

4. Severe mania...

3. High moderate mania..

2. Low moderate mania..

1. Mild mania..

O. Normal Range...

1==2==3==4==5==6==7==8==9==10==11==12==13==14==15==16==17=etc.

O. Normal Range...

1. Mild depression...

2. Low moderate depression ....

3. High moderate depression..

4. Severe depression..

Using such a chart will make your illness visible and historical to you and to your doctors. Additionally, precious time will be saved, time that can then be spent on possible drug adjustments and discussions of coping strategies. Hopefully such a record will make you a partner in deciding your course of treatment. If so, you might begin to feel that you have snatched a modicum of control back from your illness.

"The way I feel inside is not reality."

"Paranoia" is the delusion that other people know what your are thinking. It is part of bipolar disorder, undoubtedly formed from the confusion in point of view that the illness creates. For example, a lady asks me,

"Well, did you have fun last night?"

If I am in mania, I might interpret her question to be acknowledgement that I am interested in her. But if I am in depression, my interpretation might be something like,

"She knows I'm depressed. Do I wear it on my face? She's making fun of me."

The DSM IV lists six types of delusional disorders: erotomanic, grandiose, jealous, persecutory, somatic and mixed. In the fourteen years in which I was improperly medicated and/or unmedicated, I experienced the first four types for sure, and perhaps all six. In depression, I felt persecuted by my ex-wife. I felt extreme jealousy over her suitors. In mania I was driven by uncontrollable sex urges and often had grandiose ideas, such rewriting the Bible. Yet, when I got onto drugs that work for me, all of those faulty feelings disappeared...leaving me to slowly adjust to the fact that for fourteen years, "the way that I felt on the inside was not reality".

Strategies for Maintaining Relationships

Recalling and Applying Childhood Stresses

Yes, you have probably inherited a faulty limbic system, but "fossil stress" (from childhood) caused your illness to erupt. You will breakeven with your illness only when you learn to avoid or deal with (1) the fossil stress that prepared you for your illness and (2) the stress that is created by the illness itself.

In attempting to *maintain relationships*, stress caused by the illness itself must be dealt with first. You must, as it were, douse the kindled flames of your illness before you will see your relationships realistically.

The only way to do this is to rigorously follow the "Essential Behaviors" that are listed above.

It has been true for me, and I suspect that it might be true for you, that you will not be able to build new relationships until you understand the root causes of your illness. Your root causes cast long shadows that confuse your interpretation of possible new relationships. For example, because of my mother's drinking I find any woman who drinks unattractive. At the intellectual level, I understand this is a nutty attitude. Many wonderful women drink modestly. Yet my feelings are far more powerful than my thoughts, and here I am, an adult slave to my childhood stresses.

Gaining an understanding of your root stresses will require a level of honesty and psychological pain that will undoubtedly be new to you. If life has not already done it, you must remove your Previous Precious Personal Fable and replace it with a new one based upon the reality of your illness. Prior to my kindling, my personal fable was like a suit of armor. It had taken all my life to bolt together, and it was very strong. Following my kindling, it was pure Hell to peel my fable away. It was layered like an onion and it took years to reach my essence, the "real me". My reward, however, has been very great. I have broken even with a killer illness and am slowly rebuilding my life.

The process for identifying root stresses is uncomplicated, but psychologically hard.

- Work from the present to the past.
- Start with your kindling event, which will have something to do with loss of love or the threat of loss of love. With the help of your counselor and group, understand the components of your kindling event fully.
- Then search your adolescence memories, then your childhood memories, for a similar event(s). With the assistance of your counselor and group, embrace the earlier hurt, track its shadow

through the rest of your life and marvel at the pattern of behavior that it has caused you, unconsciously, to follow.

- With the assistance of your counselor and group, plot strategies for recognizing your pattern of behavior and for changing it in ways that protect your emotions.

Maintaining Adult Relationships

According to the *Handbook of Relational Diagnosis and Dysfunctional Family Patterns*[66], validated measuring instruments for testing family dysfunction exists. But as there is no agreement on which instrument to use in the emerging discipline of "Relational Diagnosis", there is no way at present to relate specific areas of family functioning to particular psychiatric illnesses. In the absence of such science, we bipolars are left to figure things out for ourselves. Here is my contribution:

- My kindling experience damaged my family relations greatly, and you may have the same problem. When I kindled, for example, I became, overnight, terrified that I was losing my mind. I stopped sleeping altogether. The experience was so profoundly different from any previous experience that I could not begin to describe or understand what was happening to me. Not only did I become mentally unhinged, my brain felt too big for my cranium. My anger was barely controllable. I spent the better part of one night standing outside the open window of my wife's romantic interest, listening to him snore and arguing with myself whether to rip through the screen and kill him. My wife, very much aware of my nightly roaming and anger, became terrified of me. At my job, I could not concentrate. I

---

66   Keitner, G.I., MD, Miller I.W., Ph.D., Ryan, C.Ec, Ph.D., (1996), "Mood Disorders and the Family", pp 434-447; See Book. Kaslow, F.W., Editor, *Handbook of Relational Diagnosis and Dysfunctional Family Patterns*, John Wiley & Sons, Inc., NYC

became convinced that my boss could "see" the confusion in my mind and would soon fire me. My wife could not understand my behaviors (no one is capable of doing so who has not experienced them). She eventually began citing my illness as a reason to divorce me. Her "betrayal" made me feel even more angry and impotent. Quickly, my self-esteem plunged from high to zero and did not recover. Quickly, I passed from anxiety over the future of my children to pathological fear. I remained at the pathological fear level until being stabilized on valproic acid, fourteen years later.

- At the other end of the spectrum, I know of others who kindled without damage to their family relationships.

- Whatever your experience with kindling, however, if you don't get on drugs that work for you, and stay on them for the rest of your life, you can kiss your family goodbye. No sane person, no mater how loving, can live with an unmedicated bipolar.

- Communication is the most important component of family life and the one most affected by bipolar disorder. It is extremely difficult to communicate whipsawing feelings and the psychoses they produce. It is extremely difficult for a metamorphosed bipolar to understand how he or she effects others.

- Trust was the first casualty in my family relations. It was very difficult for my wife to believe my version of what was happening to me.

- Anxiety is the acid of family relations and it flows freely in bipolar disorder families.

Maintaining Job Relationships

All job strategies must deal with the same three quandaries: (1) You are mentally ill and you handle stress poorly; (2) but if you admit it, you become a pariah to employers; (3) and if you get fired, your reference is toast.

Here are a few my job experiences from the fourteen years when I was unstable:

- Bosses want perfect people who can become part of a solution, not imperfect people who might add to their problems.

- If you reveal your disorder, businesses will politely lose interest in you. When I did reveal, I was always rejected, often because "I was overqualified for the job".

- If you do not reveal your disorder, business health insurers discover your hospital stays from a central clearinghouse for such information. Before they will insure you the insurers will demand an explanation for the unreported hospitalizations. If you explain, you must admit that you lied to your employer. If you don't explain, the insurer will not insure you and tell your employer. Either way, your new employer's trust in you is effected and, in my experience, your job won't last long.

- References are, of course, extremely important in securing new jobs. Because, in my unstable years, I was unable to hold jobs and I had no references at all.

- Such problems kept recurring while I was improperly medicated and I became, as a result, an extreme reactor to low levels of stress. Because such problems kept me from securing my usual kind of employment, I slowly worked my way down to jobs at the bottom of the business world, commissioned sales. Such jobs do not offer health benefits. The entire system is predicated on constantly hiring and exploiting new salespeople. Yet even a bipolar can sign on to such operations, especially when manic. Many such sales organizations are, however, run by morally ill people. Everyone gets manipulated. Territories developed get shrunk. Promising clients get taken over. Commissions earned get stolen. Those sorts of jobs are not at all the type that a stress-sensitive bipolar can cope with. Just the opposite, in fact.

Today, there are many wonderful new medicines, and no one should have to wander in a wilderness the way I did. Despite my experiences to the contrary, *lithium carbonate* is, of course, very effective for many bipolars. *Valproic acid* is very effective for even more of us. And an entirely new class of drugs, the atypical neuroleptics, might very well become the class of drugs that all of us end up on. The timing of where you are in your bipolar metamorphosis is, therefore, the most important ingredient in any job strategy. So,

- If you delay seeking treatment, kiss your present job goodbye. There is no way that an unmedicated bipolar who is beyond the kindling and intermittent reinforcement stages can perform a job.

- If you seek treatment quickly, allow 6-12 months for you and your physician to work out the course of drugs best for you. During that time you will feel awful and you will handle stress poorly. While I don't know any bipolar that was able to hold his job during his eruption period, don't give up if you are in that condition. Having a job is infinitely better than seeking a new one, and the daily routine of employment is highly therapeutic.

- Age at kindling is a major factor. An older person with bipolar disorder is far less attractive to a business than a young person with the disorder.

Finally, there is the issue of honesty with your fellow employees and business associates. Because a vast majority of people is frightened of mental illness, you must be selective in your honesty. Never volunteer what is going on. If asked, never drop the whole load. "I am being treated for a condition of the nerves" is an accurate statement that sounds far better than "I am being treated for bipolar illness".

If you do tell someone everything, be prepared to lose that person's respect. Even people who you think love you will turn away. You will become invisible. You will hurt in ways that you never thought possible.

Eventually, however, calluses will form. You will know you have them when you can say, in effect, "Here I am; this is me; take me or leave me".

Building New Relationships

Even if, like me, you blow away your family, friends and jobs during the period following kindling and before stabilization, you must replace those relationships. You will never breakeven with bipolar disorder without a support system of caring others on the outside of your ill-ness-affected thoughts and feelings. There are two stages to building new relationships: one stage is the period between kindling and stabilization, and the other one is the stage that follows stabilization.

(a) Building New Relationships After Kindling and Before Stabilization

The task of building new relationships while metamorphosing from your previous life to your new should not be underestimated. It may very well exceed your good intentions. Yet, I have done it (with many failures), and I have seen others do it.

You have read that *lithium carbonate* did not stabilize me and that my unstable period from kindling to stabilization lasted fourteen years. None, who develop bipolar disorder post 1995, when *valproic acid* was approved for the treatment of bipolar disorder, should ever have to repeat my experience. Yet, unstable periods will undoubtedly remain relatively long because the illness begins in invisibility, then extends because of denial (almost always reinforced by loved ones) and "drug non-compliance" (that is, the very harmful attitude "this drug is worse than the illness itself").

If you, like me, suddenly find yourself without caring relationships, what strategies can you follow? Here are the ones that, in hindsight, I wish I had followed:

- Upon first being diagnosed as bipolar, recognize that your relationships are at great risk.

- Tell them that you have an illness (not a "mental illness") that can be treated, but that it might take as much as six months to get your medicine right. Ask for their patience.

- Begin your drug therapy immediately.

- Keep daily charts of your moods and drug reactions for your physician.

- **NEVER** deviate from the drug prescriptions that your physician gives you, even if they make you sleep all day. Remember that it can take as long as five weeks for psychiatric drugs to become effective, and that sleep is healing to a frazzled brain.

- Begin group therapy immediately and stick with it. Don't be put off by your fellow group members. Whatever their appearance or station in life, remember that all of your fellow mentally ill will have experiences that will be helpful to you.

- Keep working as long as possible. If you lose your job, replace it with other work. Write, mow lawns, stack shelves at supermarkets, anything to keep your mind busy.

- Keep exercising. A healthy body is the reflection of a healthy mind, and vice versa.

(b) Building New Relationships after Stabilization

Following stabilization, the task of building new relationships becomes much easier. Now you are something new under the sun. Light shines from you, where previously darkness sucked. And, oddly, power will flow from your weakness. You will never be "well". Like a diabetic, you will be "contained". You will continue to have ups and down, but they will be far more gentle, and the spacing between them will be extended. You will continue to have "events", times when your memory leaves you, periods of anxiety that seemingly have no explanation, nightmares that come and go. Your sex drive may very well remain muted by your medicines. You may have to live alone for awhile. You may have a tiny amount of income. But you will know yourself. And you will understand others in ways that can't be described.

Here, in hindsight, are the things I wish I had done following my stabilization:

- If you don't already belong to one, visit churches, synagogues, mosques or temples until you find one in which you feel comfortable. Communities of worshipers are communities of caring people. Don't drop the whole load that you are a bipolar, however. Don't wear your illness on your sleeve. If someone asks, answer truthfully, with the following attitude: "This is who I am. Take me or leave me."

- If you find yourself living alone, adopt a pet. It is truly astonishing how much my Maltese and I care for each other.

- If you can't do commercial work, find and perform volunteer work. The daily routine of work is highly therapeutic.

Social Security Disability Income

If, like me, you find yourself unable to hold jobs because work stress continues to triggers mania or depression events, your next step should be job rehabilitation.

Job Rehabilitation is a social service run by the states. You will find their telephone number in the State Government section of your telephone book. Before applying, line up your referrals. They will need physician and hospital records to document your case.

Don't expect them to be magicians. You are the only expert on where you belong in the work world. You should, therefore, approach rehabilitation with some idea of what you would like to rehabilitate into. This is complicated because your illness creates poor judgement. I, for example, thought I could pull off teaching in the "peace and quite" of high school English classes. In reality, there are very few peaceful and quite high school English classes.

Therefore, I recommend this rehabilitation strategy to you:

- Those of us with BPI are born into the world as one type of person, then metamorphose into a totally new kind of person. That is, we have to give up our previous, very precious identities (businessman, nurse, "successful", "Born to Win", "gifted", "smart", "chosen", etc.) and become something new ("divorced", "unemployed", "unwanted", "mentally ill", "pariah", etc.). If your metamorphosis is not complete, that is, if you are not comfortable with what you have become, then job rehabilitation is premature.

- Obviously, you should seek to rehabilitate into jobs with low stress.

- Before deciding what type of job to rehabilitate into, discuss your ideas thoroughly with your physician(s), your group, your family and your rehabilitation specialists.

If job rehabilitation does not work for you, your next step is to apply for Social Security Disability. Social Security Disability Income has been like medicine to me. I, of course, spent fourteen years on a drug that did not stabilize me. As a result, I blew through job after job after job, earning barely enough to skim by on. Without the support of my family, I would never have survived. The anxiety that such a life produces reinforced the illness that created it. The vicious circle was broken only when I got on drugs that work that work for me, began receiving excellent counseling, and, just as importantly, began receiving a regular income from Social Security Disability.

Do not expect to qualify for SS Disability quickly, however; and unless you are truly needy, do not expect to qualify at all. I suspect that the qualification procedure moves at a snail's pace purposely. My suspicion is that such procedures were established because the preponderance of disability claims is for physical injuries, and by stretching out approval, fake claims can be identified and denied. I am certain that there are fake mental illness claims as well and that the system must be sure that it is helping truly needy people. To a truly mentally ill person, however, the process can be hellish torture.

SS: "You report that you are presently employed as an envelope stuffer. Under our rules, such employment is considered substantial and gainful."

Me: "Substantial and gainful? Can you live on minimum wages?"

SS: "You can make decisions."

Me: "Of course I can make decisions. Even schizophrenics can. The proper question is whether I make good decisions, and I defy you to review my work history and repeat that I make good decisions."

SS: "You are capable of becoming a mail room clerk."

Me: "I am mentally ill, not mentally retarded."

Now that I am finally calm, however, I look back and realize that the system was very fair and humane. It began with an application made at my local Social Security office. Then I received written instructions to visit psychologists and medical doctors, some of whom were interested in me, some of whom were suspicious of me. Then written responses to my application arrived, denying my claim and informing me of my appeal rights. When I appealed, I went through another round of visits to psychologists and doctors. Another denial of my claim resulted. I made a final claim to an Administrative Judge. At that level, I finally get to deal with a person, not letter-writers. I could have hired a lawyer at any step in the process, and he or she would have represented me for a contingency fee of 20% to 33% of my eventual settlement. I never hired a lawyer. I chose to trust the judge. Because I did, I got to keep 100% of my award.

In summary, I recommend this strategy to you:

- If job rehabilitation fails for you, file your Social Security Disability claim as soon as possible. If you subsequently win an award, you will receive back pay to the date of your original filing.

- Do not get discouraged by the early trips to Social Security's independent doctors, or by the early denials of your claim. Stay the course.

- Trust the system and never be disrespectful to any Social Security employee. I have found them, and all the rest of the safety net employees to be truly caring people. Yes, the system as a whole is bureaucratic and frustrating in the extreme. But the people who work within it are not. Often, they are as frustrated as the rest of us.

The Behavioral Goal

Any model for breaking even with affective illness must include a strategy for dealing with the vast majority of your acquaintances (including doctors, ministers, rabbis, and priests) who are going to say, "Well, now that you understand it, snap out of it!" As politely as possible, tell those ignorant people these things:

- That your neuronal pathways have been trained since childhood to behave a certain way.

- That your neuronal pathways are invisible, they can't be felt like an arm or a leg, and that understanding them is more complicated than understanding space physics.

- That the way your brain has memorized your illness is unknown and is likely to remain that way.

- That the best you can do is to live your life forward while understanding it backward.
- That you are a chemically unique person and if they don't like you the way you are, they can lump it!

About the Author

Michael Crawford graduated from the University of Houston in 1961. He had a career in educational publishing until 1981 when he kindled into "Bipolar II" mental illness. Today he lives alone, writes and substitute teaches. He has three children, one grandchild and a bossy Maltese named "Barkley".

Annotated Bibliography

1. Alper, J.S. & Natowicz, M.R., (1993). On establishing the genetic basis of mental disease. *Trends-Neuroscience: 16, 19*: 387-389.

Abstract: Many of the recent studies reporting genetic linkages for mental illnesses such as schizophrenia and manic-depression have been retracted. The authors of this article argue that the fundamental reason for the difficulties in this research field lies in the strongly held preconceived belief that the primary cause of these illnesses is in fact genetic. All scientists hold preconceived ideas. However, such ideas are more likely to result in erroneous conclusions in the study of human behavior than in other more 'objective' research areas. Moreover, it is especially important that researchers studying human behavior be aware of their biases and learn to compensate for them because of the social consequences of their work.

2. Baron, M., (1991). X-linkage and manic-depressive illness: a reassessment. *Soc.-Biol. 38, 3-4:* 179-188.

Abstract: Genetic-epidemilogical data and linkage studies with chromosomal markers are reviewed from the vantage point of X-linked inheritance. The results overall suggest that a gene predisposing to manic-depression (bipolar affective illness) localized on the X-chromosome may exist in a subgroup of bipolar cases. However, in light of conflicting findings and methodological uncertainties in studying a disorder with unclear phenotype and complex inheritance, this issue is not yet closed. Additional research, including new linkage data and extension and re-evaluation of published data is required to further our understanding of this intriguing hypothesis.

3. Barnett, S. A., 1998. *The Science of Life.* Allen & Unwin, St. Leonards 2065 Australia.

4. Baumann, B. & Bogerts, B., 1999. The pathomorphology of schizophrenia and mood disorders: similarities and differences. *Schizophr Res* Sep 29; 39(2): 141-8.

Abstract: In this article, post-mortem neurohistological and structural imaging studies of schizophrenia and mood disorders are briefly reviewed; In contrast to the large number of post-mortem studies on schizophrenia published during the last 20 years, very few histological studies of affective disorders are available. After commenting on CT and MRI studies, as well as on neuropathological findings on whole-brain size, cortex, frontal and temporal lobes, limbic system, basal ganglia, thalamus, brain stem and cortical asymmetry, it is concluded that despite a broad overlap in structural findings in the so-called endogenous psychoses, heteromodal association cortex, limbic system and structural asymmetry are more affected in schizophrenia while subtle structural abnormalities in the basal ganglia, especially in the nucleus accumbens and in hypothalamic areas, might play a crucial role in mood disorders.

5. Berrettini, W.H., 2000. Susceptibility loci for bipolar disorder: overlap with inherited vulnerability to schizophrenia. *Biological Psychiatry*, February 1; 47(3): 245-51

Abstract: Genetic epidemiological studies reveal that relatives of bipolar probands are at increased risk for recurrent unipolar, bipolar, and schizoaffective disorders, whereas relatives of probands with schizophrenia are at increased for sschizophrenia, schizoaffective, and recurrent unipolar disorders. The overlap in familial risk may reflect shared genetic susceptibility. Recent genetic linkage studies have defined confirmed susceptibility loci for BPI disorder for multiple regions of the human genome, including 4p16, 12q24, 18p11.2, 18q22, 21q21, 22q11-13, and Xq26. Studies of schizophrenia kindred have yielded robust evidence for susceptibility at 18p11.2 and 22q11-13, both of which are implicate in susceptibility to BPI disorder. Similarly, confirmed schizophrenia vulnerability loci have been mapped for 6p24, 8p and 13q32. Strong statistical evidence for a 13q32 BPI susceptibility locus has been reported. Thus, both family and molecular studies of these disorders suggest shared genetic susceptibility. These two groups of disorders may not be so distinct as current [classification] suggests

6. Brodley, B.T., (1986) "Client-Centered Therapy, What Is It? What Is It Not?", paper presented at the Association for the Development of Person-Centered Approach, University of Chicago, September 3-7.

7. Brown, R., (1989). U.S. experience with valproate in manic depressive illness: a multicenter trial. *Journal of Clinical Psychiatry 50, [3, Suppl]:* 13-16

Abstract: Valproic acid and its enteric-coated derivative, divalproex sodium, have been used extensively in a wide variety of seizure disorders. Recent preliminary research demonstrated the effectiveness of valproate in the treatment of manic-depressive illness, including acute mania, prevention of bipolar episodes, and schizoaffective disorder. In uncontrolled and controlled studies, treatment-resistant patients with these disorders have responded well to valproate. Preliminary results of an ongoing community-based open trial of valproate treatment of those affective illnesses reveal that valproate is frequently effective and has a favorable side effect profile. Overall, approximately two out of three patients with refractory bipolar disorder respond to acute therapy with valproate. Response in schizoaffective patients has been moderate, and valproate seems to be less effective in the treatment of depression. Experience suggests the importance of monitoring plasma drug levels to maximize efficacy and minimize potential toxicity.

8. Cahill, L.; McGaugh, J.L., (1998. Mechanisms of emotional arousal and lasting declarative memory. *Trends in Neurosciences, 21 (7):* 294-9.

Abstract: Neuroscience is witnessing growing interest in understanding brain mechanisms of memory formation for emotionally arousing events, a development closely related to renewed interest in the concept of memory consolidation. Extensive research in animals implicates stress hormones and the amygdaloid complex as key, interacting modulators of memory consolidation for emotional events. Considerable evidence suggests that the amygdala is not a site of long-term explicit or declarative memory storage, but serves to influence memory-storage processes in other brain regions, such as the hippocampus, striatum and neocortex. Human-subject studies confirm the prediction of animal work that the amygdala is involved with the formation of enhanced declarative memory for emotionally arousing events.

9. Citrome, L.; Levine, J.; & Allingham, B. (1998). Utilization of valproate: Extent of inpatient use in the New York State Office of Mental Health. *Psychiatric Quarterly, 69, 4:* 283-300.

Abstract: A database containing patient and drug prescription information for every in-patient in the adult civil facilities of the New York State Office of Mental Health was queried. In 1994, 2,888 of 18,668 patients received valproate. In 1996, 4,247 of 12,444 patients received valproate. In 1996, approximately 50% of all patients diagnosed as bipolar or schizoaffective, and 28% of all patents diagnosed with schizophrenia, received valproate. Once on valproate, over 90% remained on it after 2 weeks, with no difference found in the discontinuation rates between valproic acid or divalproex sodium at the end of the initial 14 day period. Patients received valproate for approximately two-thirds of their hospital stay, at a mean dose of 1400 mg/day. 95% also received concomitant antipsychotics, and 20% received concomitant lithium. Use of lithium and carbamazepine was less in 1996 than in 1994, but the magnitude of this change was much less than the increase in use of valproate. From 1994 to 1996, valproate use has more than doubled, and it is being used widely in patients with schizophrenia, and off-label indication for which there is only anecdotal support in the literature. Given the lack of difference in early discontinuation rates, there are probably no dramatic differences in side effects for the two preparations of valproate.

10. *Diagnostic and Statistical Manual of Mental Disorders, Forth Edition.* (1994). Washington DC, American Psychiatric Association.

11. Ewald, H.: Mors, O.; Koed, K.; Eiberg, H.; Kruse, T.A., (1997). Susceptibility loci for bipolar affective disorder on chromosome 18? A review and study of Danish families. *Psychiatric-Genetics 7, 1:* 1-12.

Abstract: Chromosome 18 is one of the most promising chromosomes in the search for susceptibility genes for bipolar disorder based on results from cytogenetic, linkage, and association studies. Susceptibility loci on chromosome 18p and 18q have bee suggested for bipolar affective disorder. The authors present a review of published studies which suggests that it is presently unclear whether one or more susceptibility loci on chromosome 18 exist, and that their more accurate localization is unknown. The present study investigated 27 DNA markers on chromosome 18 in two Danish families with bipolar affective disorder. Positive lod scores were found in the larger family for markers on chromosome 18q12, especially for the affection status model which only includes bipolar patients. Thee highest lod score found was for marker D 18S67, 1.83 at 0.05 recombination fraction. ((c) 1998 APA/PsycINFO, all rights reserved).

12. Federal Drug Administration Home Page (1998, December). Available: *www.fda.gov/fdahomepage.html*

13. Gershon, E.S.; Badner, J.A.; Goldin, L.R.; Sanders, A.R.; Cravchik, A.; Detera, W.; Sevilla, D., (1998). Closing in on genes for manic-depressive illness and schizophrenia. *Neuropsychopharmacology 18, 4*: 233-242.

Abstract: Advances in the human genetic map and in genetic analysis of linkage and association in complex inheritance traits have led to genetic progress in thee major psychoses. For chromosome 6 in schizophrenia and for chromosomes 18 and 21 in manic-depressive illness, there are reports of linkage in several independent data sets. These are small effect genes, best detected with affected-relative-pair linkage methods. Association with candidate genes is an alternative strategy to uncovering susceptibility genes for these illnesses, but convincing associations remain to be demonstrated. New clinical and laboratory investigation methods are being developed. Testing every gene in the human genome for association with illness has recently be proposed (N. Risch and K. Merikangas, 1996). This would require further progress in characterizing the genome and in automated large-scale genotyping. The best type of pedigree sampling for common disease studies, whether for linkage or association, is not yet established. An endophenotype hybrid strategy can combine genetic linkage, association, and pathophysiologic studies. As clinical molecular investigation methods advance, identification of disease susceptibility, mutations and delineation of their pathophysiological roles may be expected. ((c) 1998 APA/PsycINFO, all rights reserved).

14. Gershon, E.S., (1989). Recent developments in genetics of manic-depressive illness. *Journal of Clinical Psychiatry 50, [12 Suppl]:* 4-7.

Abstract: Bipolar affective disorder appears to be a heterogeneous disorder with multiple independently inherited disease genes, each giving similar clinical results (bipolar, unipolar, and other disorders). This conclusion derives from the recent findings of separate forms of illness linked to single gene markers, with the preponderance of cases in several studies not linked to any of them. At this time, reports of linkage to chromosome 11 and to the color-blindness region of X chromosome are widely accepted, but reports of linkage of the HLA region of chromosome 6 have been criticized and are considered controversial. Persons born in successive decades of the 20th century have progressively greater risks for bipolar and unipolar affective disorders, suicide, and alcoholism, but not schizophrenia. This multinational trend begins with persons born in the 1930's and extends to the present time (or possible until the present decade). For affective disorders, this trend has greater effect in families of affective disorder patients than in the population as a whole, implying a genetic-environment interaction.

15. Ghaemi, S.N.; Boiman, E.E.; Goodwin, F.K. (1999). Kindling and second messengers: an approach to the neurobiology of recurrence in bipolar disorder. *Biological Psychiatry, 45 (2):* 137-44.

Abstract: Since bipolar disorder is inherently a longitudinal illness characterized by recurrence and cycling of mood episodes, neurobiological theories involving kindlinglike phenomena appear to possess a certain explanatory power. An approach to understanding kindlinglike phenomena at the molecular level has been made possible by advances in research on second-messenger systems in the brain. The time frame of interest has shifted from the microseconds of presynaptic events to hours, days, months, and even years in the longer duration of events beyond the synapse–through second messengers, gene regulation, and synthesis of long-acting trophic factors. These complex interlocking systems may explain how environmental stress could interact over time with genetic vulnerability to produce illness. In its two sections, this paper will review an approach to understanding two major aspects of the neurobiology of bipolar disorder: kindling phenomena and second-messenger mechanisms. We will suggest that these two fields of research together help explain the biology of recurrence.

16. Ghaemi, A.N.; Stoll, A.L.; Pope, H.G. (1995). Lack of insight in bipolar disorder. *The Journal of Nervous and Mental Disease, 183, 7:* 464-467.

Abstract: This study examined the clinical correlates of lack of insight in bipolar disorder. In 28 acutely manic patients interviewed upon hospitalization and/or discharge, mean scores on the Insight and Treatment Attitudes Questionnaire (ITAQ) improved only slightly, from 12.0 on admission to 15.5 on discharge (p = .08), despite marked improvement in other psychiatric symptoms. A reciprocal relationship was found between higher ITAQ scores and involuntary hospitalization (r = -.38). Like schizophrenia, bipolar disorder appears to be a condition in which poor insight is a prominent characteristic.

17. Goddard, G.V.; McIntyre, D.C. & Leech, C.K. (1969). A permanent change in brain function resulting from daily electrical stimulation. *Experimental Neurology 25:* 295-330.

Abstract: Brief burst of nonpolarizing electrical brain stimulation were presented once each day at constant intensity. At first the stimulation had little effect on behavior and did not cause electrographic after-discharge. With repetition the response to stimulation progressively changed to include localized seizure discharge, behavioral automatisms and eventually, bilateral clonic convulsions. Thereafter, the animal responded to each daily burst of stimulation with a complete convulsion. The effect was obtained from bipolar stimulation of loci associated with the limbic system, but not from stimulation of many other regions of the brain. Parametric studies and control observations revealed that the effect was due to electrical activation and not to tissue damage, poison, edema, or gliosis. The changes in brain function were shown to be both permanent and trans-synaptic in nature. Massed-trial stimulation, with short inter-burst intervals, rarely led to convulsions. The number of stimulation trials necessary to elicit the first convulsion decreased as the interval between trials approached 24 hours. Further increase in the into-trial interval had little effect on the number of trials to first convulsion. High-intensity stimulation studies revealed that the development of convulsions was not based simply on threshold reduction, but involved complex reorganization of function. Experiments with two electrodes in separate parts of the limbic system revealed that previously established convulsions could facilitate the establishment of a second convulsive focus, but that the establishment of this second convulsive focus partially suppressed the otherwise permanent convulsive properties of the original focus. **From page 328:** There is a remarkable similarity between many properties of the kindling effect and properties of normal learning. For example, each is a relatively permanent change resulting from repeated experience, the limbic system is implicated in both kindling and learning, both involve trans-synapic changes in function, both demonstrate positive transfer from one stimulus to another, and in both cases the acquisition of a new response results in retroactive interference with old responses. These arguments, of course, are based entirely on analogy and are speculative.

18. Goodwin, F.K., (1989). The biology of recurrence: New directions for the pharmacologic bridge. *Journal of Clinical Psychiatry 50, [12, Suppl]*: 40-44.

Abstract: Recurrence is a fundamental reality of the major affective disorders and must be considered in treatment planning. Historically, however, information regarding the pathophysiology and neurobiology of affective disorders was not gained from studies on recurrence, but rather from research unitizing drugs classified on the basis of their effect on acute manic and/or depressive states. Though such cross-sectional strategies were critical in developing the original amine hypotheses, they also were inherently limited. Today, accumulating information regarding differential drug effects on cycle length calls for reexamining the pharmacologic bridge from the perspective of the nascent neurobiology of recurrence of affective disorders. This presentation considers the array of drugs now used in treating mood disorders and reviews recent data relating to the role of acute and maintenance treatments on the occurrence of manic and hypomanic reactions in bipolar patients. In addition, emerging data on the impact of longitudinal treatments on the natural course of bipolar illness are used to develop a model for examining the effects of treatment on recurring unipolar illness.

19. Guthrie, W.K.C., (1960). *The Greek Philosophers.* Harper Torchbooks, NYC.

20. Guze, B.H. & Gitlin, M. (1994) The Neuropathologic basis of major affective disorders: neuroanatomic insights. *Journal of Neuropsychiatry 6 (2):* 114-121

Abstract: Attempts to elucidate the pathophysiology of symptom production in mood disorders can be enhanced by information from two sources. First, insights in localization can be gained from the secondary mood disorders; these clinical problems suggest the brain regions that, when altered, are associated with specific symptoms. Second, both structural and functional brain imaging suggest specific regions where abnormalities are associated with mood disorders. Data that emerge from these sources implicate the basal ganglia, frontal cortex and temporal lobes in the production of mood disorder symptoms.

However, the specific neuroanatomic subregions involved and the associated biochemical changes await full elucidation.

21. Keitner, G.I., MD, Miller I.W., Ph.D., Ryan, C.Ec, Ph.D., (1996), "Mood Disorders and the Family", pp 434-447; **See Book.** Kaslow, F.W., Editor, *Handbook of Relational Diagnosis and Dysfunctional Family Patterns* (1996), John Wiley & Sons, Inc., NYC

22. Kraepelin E.. *Manic-Depressive Insanity and Paranoia.* Translated by Barclay, R.M., edited by Robertson, G.M.,. Edinburgh, E.&S. Livingstone, 1921.

23. Kwok, J.B.; Adams, L.J.; Salmon, J.A.; Mitchell, P.B.; Schofield, P.R. (1999). Nonparametric stimulation-based statistical analyses for bipolar affective disorder locus on chromosome 21q22.3. *American Journal of Medical Genetics. 88 (1):* 99-102.

Abstract: Straub et al. [1994: Nat Genet 8:291-296] reported a candidate bipolar affective disorder (BAD) locus on chromosome 21q22.3. As a replication study, we analyzed 12 Australian BAD pedigrees for the presence of excess allele sharing and cosegregation with the putative chromosome 21q22.3 BAD locus, using six microsatellite markers...This report provides additional support for the suggestive linkage of a susceptibility locus for BAD on chromosome 21q22.3.

24. Leverich, G.S., & Post, R.M., (1998). Life Charting of Affective Disorders. *The International Journal of Neuropsychiatric Medicine 3 (5):* 21-37.

Abstract: The recurrent and frequently chronic course of affective disorders requires careful delineation of the number, frequency, and pattern of prior and current episodes and their response to pharmacotherapies and to help develop optimal assessment and treatment approaches for these potentially lethal medical illnesses. To better track and monitor the longitudinal course of unipolar and bipolar illness and to promote more effective management, we developed the retrospective and prospective National Institute of Mental Health Life Chart Methodology (NIMH-LCM). The principles of retrospective and prospective life charting are the focus of this article. Following introductory back-ground information on affective disorders, the influence of Kraepelin's work and his use of life charts are reviewed as the basis and framework for the MIMH-LCM. The use of life charting both retrospectively and prospectively is discussed, with examples of its utility and benefits.

25. MacKinnon, D.F.; Jamison, Kay Redfield; DePaulo, J.R., (1997). Genetics of manic depressive illness. *Annual Review of Neuroscience 20*: 355-373.

Abstract: States that manic depressive illness (MDI) is a common and frequently debilitating familial bipolar psychiatric disorder. Efforts to understand the mechanisms of inheritance have been hindered by the complexity of the phenotype, which may range from benign mood swings to chronic psychosis, and by apparently nonmendelian modes of transmission. Early reports of linkage to chromosomal loci have fallen into doubt; however then have helped encourage the development of more sophisticated methods for analyzing complex phenotypes. Using such methods, linkage of MDI to loci on chromosome 18 has been reported and apparently replicated, and work is proceeding to identify genes associated with what is probably a genetically heterogeneous set of disorders. Molecular mechanisms of inheritance are elucidated. It will be important to consider the ethical implications of genetic testing in a clinically and genetically complex disorder such as MDI. ((c) 1998 APA/PsycINFO, all rights reserved).

26. McGaugh, J. L.; Bermudez-Rattoni, F.; Prado-Alcala, R. A., (1995). *Plasticity In The Central Nervous System, Learning and Memory.* Lawrence Erlbaum Associates, Publishers, Mahwah, New Jersey.

27. Martin, A. (1998). Psychoparmacology update: What's new in the treatment of depression. *Psychoanalysis and Psychotherapy 15, 1:* 131-134.

Abstract: This paper provides and update on the pharmacological treatment of depression. Over the last decade, the field of antidepressant treatments had improved remarkably in regards to the quality and quantity of available options to help people who are depressed and who may have ancillary symptoms that often accompany depression (e.g., obsessiveness, anxiety, anger, or irritability) or who have personality characteristics that predispose a person to become depressed (e.g., dysthymia or borderline personality features). During the 10 years since Prozac became available in 1987, new antidepressants have been released at the rate of about 1 per year. These newer antidepressants have been more tolerable (i.e., less side effects, overall) and safer (e.g., less serious side effects, including being much less dangerous if taken in an overdose) while being at least as efficacious as the older antidepressants and the MAO inhibitors. ((c) 1998 APA/PsycINFO, all rights reserved).

28. "Psychotherapy," *Microsoft® Encarta® Encyclopedia 99.* © 1993-1998 Microsoft Corporation. All rights reserved.

29. Monroe, Russell R., *Creative Brainstorms,* ©1992, Irvington Publishers, Inc. New York, New York

30. Nothen, M.M.; Chchon, S. Rohleder, H.; Hemmer, S.; Franzek, E.; Fritze, J.; Albus, M.; Borrmann-Hassenbach, M.; Kreiner, R.; Weigelt, B.; Minges, J.; Lichermann, D.; Maier, W.; Craddock, N.; Frimmers, R.;

Holler, T.; Baur, M.P.; Rietchel, M.; Propping, P. (1999). *Molecular Psychiatry, 4 (1):* 76-84.

Abstract: Previous reported linkage of bipolar affective disorder to DNA markers on chromosome 18 was reexamined in a large sample of German bipolar families. Twenty-three short tandem repeat markers were investigated in 57 families containing 103 individuals with bipolar I disorder (BPI), 26 with bipolar II disorder (BPII), nine with schizoaffective disorder of the bipolar type (SA/BP), and 38 individuals with recurrent unipolar depression (UPR). Evidence for linkage was tested with parametric and non-parametric methods under two definitions of the affected phenotype. Analysis of the 57 families revealed no robust evidence for linkage. Following previous reports, we performed separate analyses after subdividing the families with respect to the sex of the transmitting parent. Fourteen families were classified as paternal and 12 families as maternal. In 31 families, the parental lineage of transmission of the disease could not be determines ('either' families). Evidence for linkage was obtained for chromosomal region 18p11.2 in the paternal families and for 18q22-23 in the 'either' families. The findings on 18p11.2 and 18q22-23 support prior evidence for susceptibility loci in these regions. The parent-of-origin effect on 18p22-23 is confirmed in our sample. The delineation of characteristics of 'either' families requires further study.

31. *On-line Medical Dictionary, http://www.graylab.ac.uk/omd/index.html.*

32. Post, R.M., 1999. Comparative pharmacology of bipolar disorder and schizophrenia. *Schizophr Res Sep 29*; 39(2):153-8; discussion 163

Abstract: The treatment of acute mania and schizophrenia overlap considerably in terms of the typical and atypical neuroleptics, but begin to diverge with the recognized mood stabilizers for bipolar affective illness–lithium, carbamazepine, and valproate–which are substantially less effective in schizophrenia than in affective illness. Moreover, the L-type calcium channel blocker, verapamil, is reported to be effective in mania, but it may exacerbate schizophrenia. A series of new putative mood stabilizing anticonvulsants (such as lamotrigine, gabapentin, and topiramate) and possible second-messenger targeted treatments (tamoxifen and omega-3 fatty acids) deserve further study in both affective and schizophrenic syndromes. Repeated transcranial magnetic stimulation (rTMS) of the brain offers considerable promise in the treatment of a variety of neuropsychiatric syndromes, especially with preliminary evidence of frequency-dependent effects on regional cerebral blood flow. New insights about the potential neurotrophic effects of lithium and the gene transcriptional effects of other psychotropics offer exciting new targets for therapeutics and strategies for future clinical trials and therapeutic applications in both syndromes.

33. Post, R.M.; Frye, M.A.; Denicoff, K.D.; Leverich, G.S.; Kimbrell, T.A.; & Denn, R.T. (1998). Beyond lithium in the treatment of bipolar illness. *Neuropsychopharmacology 19, 3*: 206-219.

Abstract: Dramatic changes have recently occurred in the availability of treatment options for bipolar illness. Second generation mood stabilizing anticonvulsants, carbamazepine and valproate, are now widely used as alternatives or adjuncts to lithium. High potency benzodiazepines are also used as alternatives to typical neuroleptics, and now atypical neuroleptics are demonstrating efficacy and better side effect profiles than the typicals. Thyroid augmentation strategies and dihydropyridine L-type calcium channel blockers require further clinical trials to define their role. Putative third generation mood stabilizing anticonvulsants, lamotrigine, gabapentin and topiramate, have unique mechanisms of action and deserve further systematic study, as does the potential role for nonconvulsive brain stimulation with repeated transcranial magnetic stimulation (rTMS). These and a host of other potential treatment options now require a new generation of clinical trials to help identify clinical and biological markers of response and optimal use alone and in complex combination therapeutic regimens. ((c) 1998 APA/PsycINFO, all rights reserved)(journal abstract).

34. Post, R.M.; Frye, M.A.; Gabriele, S.L.; Denikoff, K.D. (1998). The Role of Complex Combination Therapy in the Treatment of Refractory Bipolar Illness. *The International Journal of Neuropsychiatric Medicine 3*, 5: 66-86.

Abstract: In this article, we present rationales for using complex combination therapy therapeutic approach. We review a case example of successful remission that was achievable only with complex combination therapy, and examine it theoretical implications. Practical approaches to devising the optimal complex combination treatment for individual patients are explained, and we look to the development of new methodologies and a more systematic database for decision making in the future. **From The Introduction:** Many of the issues related to the acute and long-term approaches to the refractory bipolar patient emanate from a fundamental reconceptualization of the illness. It is now apparent that it is a recurrent, potentially incapacitating and lethal medical illness associated with physiological and biochemical abnormalities in the brain and the somatic and endocrine systems. There is also considerable evidence that the illness does not remain static and is highly pleomorphic [the occurrence of more than one distinct form in the life cycle of the illness] over time. **From Theoretical Implications:** This psychological and neurobiological battlefield would appear to take place on multiple levels of neural adaptation, including at the level of gene expression, and one could conceptualize this process as a battle with a universe of forces leading to illness continuously needing to be held in check. In some individuals with either lesser degrees of genetic or experiential vulnerability, or increased degrees of social support and increased resiliency and strength of endogenous adaptive factors, this may be relatively easy to achieve with careful maintenance of lithium or other mood stabilizer monotherapy. / However, when this desired outcome is not possible, more complex, multimodal psychopharmacological and psychological approaches are required in order to maintain even moderate mood stability. It is, perhaps, under added pressures that drive illness pathology (such as comorbid alcohol or substance abuse, repeated exploration of the futility of drug discontinuation during hypomanic or manic episodes, lack of social support compounded by illness-driven losses of family, economic, and social supports) that sustained responsivity may be more tenuous and breakthrough episodes occur. In our model of tolerance development, we can manipulate the driving force of the illness by increasing the intensity of the amygdala stimulation to full-blown kindled seizures. In this and other instances of higher compare d with lower illness drive, tolerance or breakthrough seizures (first occurring intermittently and then progressing to a complete loss of efficacy) develop much more rapidly. In a similar fashion, we would postulate in affective illness that for those with increased genetic and experiential risk factors (as well as greater number of prior episodes; a later stage of illness presentation; and a more complex manifestation of illness cyclicity with either continuous rhythmic cycling or dysrhythmic ["dys" = "impaired"] and ultradian cycling [cycles greater than once per week], more heroic pharmacotherapeutic measures would become necessary. In these types of instances of postulated high illness drive, the question emerges as to how to approach the required complex psychopharmacology in the most rational way possible for individual patients in the absence of systematic clinical trials literature to guide threapeutics.

35. Post, R. M. & Weiss, S.R.B., (1998). Sensitization and Kindling Phenomena in Mood, Anxiety, and Obsessive-Compulsive Disorders:

The Role of Serotonergic Mechanisms in Illness Progression. *Biological Psychiatry, 44*: 193-206

Abstract: A number of untreated or inadequately treated psychiatric illness often demonstrate syndrome progression manifested by either increasing frequency, severity, or spontaneity of episodes. Behavioral sensitization to psychomotor stimulants (and its cross sensitization to stress) and electrophysiological kindling provide two very different models for conceptualizing physiological and behavioral abnormalities that progress in severity in response to the same inducing stimulation over time. These models are highly indirect and the behaviors induced with specific pharmacologic interventions do not directly parallel those in many of these psychiatric syndromes. Nonetheless, the preclinical models help us conceptualize potential mechanisms involved in syndrome progression based on experience-dependent modifications of the genome at the level of transcriptional regulation. In both preclinical models, agents that are effective in the earlier developmental phase of sensitization or kindling are not necessarily effective in amelioration of the full-blown syndromes, and vice versa. Thus, these models also suggest a variety of intervention principles that can be directly tested in the clinic, such as differential efficacy of treatments a function of stage of evolution of the given syndrome. Although serotonergic mechanisms do not appear central to the basic phenomena of sensitization and kindling, they appear capable of modulating their development and severity. As such, it becomes of considerable importance to assess whether serotonergic mechanisms that have been implicated in acute treatment of mood and anxiety syndromes are also involved in the longitudinal course and prevention of syndrome progression or occurrence. Identification of the more precise molecular mechanisms involved might provide a target for new therapeutic approaches to these recurrent and potentially disabling major psychiatric illnesses.

36. Post, R.M., Denicoff, K.D., Frye, M.A., Dunn, R.T., Leverich, C.S., Osuch, E., Speer, A. 1998. A history of the use of anticonvulsants as mood stabilizers in the last two decades of the 20th century. *Neuropsycobiplogy Oct; 38(3): 152-66.*

Abstract: Anticonvulsants have moved into an important position as alternatives and adjuncts to lithium carbonate in the treatment of bipolar illness. Work with the nonhomologous model of kindled seizures helped in the choice of carbamazepine as a potential mood stabilizer and in the study of the mechanisms of action of the second generation anticonvulsants carbamazepine and valproate, as well as the putative third generation psychotropic anticonvulsants lamatrigine and gabepentin. Anticonvulsant neuropeptides such as TRH and nonconvulsant approaches with repeated transcranial magnetic stimulation (rTMS) also appear promising.

37. Post, R.M.; Ketter, T.A.; Denicoff, P.J; Pazzaglia, P.J.; Leverich, G.S.; Marangell, L.B.; Callahan, A.M.; George, M.S.; Frye, M.A., (1996). The place of anticonvulsant therapy in bipolar illness. *Psychopharmacology 128:* 115-129.

Abstract: With the increasing recognition of lithium's inadequacy as an acute and prophylactic treatment for many patients and subtypes of bipolar illness, the search for alternative agents has centered around the mood stabilizing anticonvulsants, carbamazepine and valproate. In many instances, these drugs are effective alone or in combination with lithium in those patients less responsive to lithium monotherapy (including those with greater numbers of prior episodes, rapid-cycling, dysphoric mania, co-morbid substance abuse or other associated medical problems), and patients without a family history of bipolar illness in first-degree relatives. Nineteen double-blind studies utilizing a variety of designs suggest that carbamazepine, or its keto-congener, oxcarbazepine, is effective in acute mania; six controlled studies report evidence of the efficacy of valproate in the treatment of acute mania as well. Fourteen controlled or partially controlled studies of prophylaxis suggest carbamazepine is also effective in preventing both manic and depressive episodes. Valproate prophylaxis data, although based entirely on uncontrolled studies, appear equally promising. Thus, both drugs are widely used and are now recognized as major therapeutic tools for lithium-nonresponsive bipolar illness. The high-potency anticonvulsant benzodiazepines, clonazepam and lorazepam, are used adjunctively with lithium or the anticonvulsant mood stabilizers as substitutes or alternatives for neuroleptics in the treatment of manic breakthroughs. Preliminary controlled clinical trials suggest that the calcium channel blockers may have antimanic or mood-stabilizing effects in a subgroup of patients. A new series of anticonvulsants has just been FDA-approved and warrant clinical trials to determine their efficacy in acute and long-term treatment of mania and depression. Systematic exploration of the optimal use of lithium and the mood-stabilizing anticonvulsants alone and in combination, as well as with adjunctive antidepressants, is now required so that more definitive treatment recommendations for different types and stages of bipolar illness can be more strongly evidence based.

38. Post, R.M.; Ketter, T.A.; Pazzaglia, P.J.; Denicoff, K.; George, M. S.; Callahan, A.; Leverich, G.; Fry, M., (1996). Rational polypharmacy in the bipolar affective disorders. *Epilepsy-Res-Suppl., 11:* 153-80.

Abstract: Bipolar affective illness represents a syndrome not readily treated by a single agent. Approximately 50% of patients are inadequately responsive to lithium and the majority of patients require supplemental antidepressants, antimanic, antipsychotic or hypnotic medications. These traditional adjunctive medications are associated with potential problems. Antidepressants may precipitate mania (at a rate about double that of placebo) or cause cycle acceleration. Neuroleptics may be associated with either more profound or longer depressive phases, and clearly increase the risk of tardive dyskinesia, to which bipolar patients appear particularly predisposed. Moreover, there are subgroups of patients who are known to be poorly responsive to lithium. These include patients with rapid cycling, dysphoric mania, co-morbid drug or alcohol abuse, a pattern of depression-mania-well interval (D-M-I, as opposed to the M-D-I pattern), and patients without a family history of bipolar illness in first-degree relatives. There is increasing recognition that the anticonvulsants, carbamazepine and valproate, are effective alternatives or adjuncts to lithium in the acute and long-term treatment of bipolar illness. Ideally, one would want to assess whether patients who were unresponsive to lithium were responsive to an anticonvulsant alone prior to utilizing lithium in addition to anticonvulsant combination therapy. However, from the clinical perspective, it is often more expedient to use an anticonvulsant adjunctively to lithium to assess the efficacy of this combination and establish mood stabilization. When lithium is not discontinued, the increased morbidity during lithium withdrawal also would not occur and would not confound the evaluation of the new agent. We suggest the initial use of acute adjuncts to lithium with the anticonvulsants carbamazepine or valproate (instead of neuroleptics) so that their efficacy can be assessed in the individual's acute episode, with the likelihood of a positive response in longer-term prophylaxis. Hypnotic benzodiazepines with anticonvulsant properties, such as clonazepam or lorazepam, are often used to help induce sleep in escalating bipolar patients, and may be useful adjuncts as well. Patients who were inadequately responsive to either carbamazepine or valproate alone may be responsive to the anticonvulsant combination. In a similar fashion, one can also utilize several mood-stabilizing drugs (lithium and an anticonvulsant, such as carbamazepine or valproate,) in the treatment of depressive breakthroughs, and then augment this combination (if necessary) with a catecholamine-active antidepressant, such as bupropion, or a serotonin-selective reuptake inhibitor (SSRI), such as fluoxetine, paroxetine, sertraline, or, if necessary, a monoamine oxidase inhibitor (MAOI). Once the patient has responded to a combination of drugs, it becomes problematic to decide whether the last agent added was the crucial ingredient in helping the patient achieve remission, or whether that remission might have occurred with this agent alone. A conservative approach would have merit in patients who are finally stabilized on complex polypharmacy regimens only after many years of sequential trials; in this instance, the potential risk of re-exacerbating the illness with a taper of one of the drugs in the regimen. Rational polypharmacy should, thus, be implemented with careful delineation of the prior course of illness (typically using life chart methodology) and targeted treatment outcomes titrated against side effects, using sequential clinical trials in individual patients who have not adequately responded to monotherapy. In this fashion, it is hoped that pharmacodynamic differences among agents can be maximized and pharmacokinetic and side effects minimized.

39. Post, R.M. & Weiss, S.R., (1996). A speculative model of affective illness cyclicity based on patterns of drug tolerance observed in amygdala-kindled seizures. *Mol-Neurobiol., 1996 Aug; 13(1):* 33-60.

Abstract: Under certain circumstances, amygdala-kindled animals that were initially drug responsive can develop highly individualized patterns of seizure breakthroughs progressing toward a complete loss of drug efficacy. This initial drug efficacy may reflect the combination of drug-related exogenous neurochemical mechanisms and illness-induced endogenous compensatory mechanisms. However, we postulate that when seizures are inhibited, the endogenous illness-induced adaptations dissipate (the "time-off seizure" effect), leading the re-emergence of seizures, a re-induction of a new, but diminished, set of endogenous compensatory mechanisms, and a temporary period of renewed drug efficacy. At the pattern repeats, an intermittent or cyclic response to the anticonvulsant treatment emerges, leading toward complete drug tolerance. We also postulate that the cyclic pattern accelerates over time because of both the failure of robust illness-induced endogenous adaptations to emerge and the progression in pathophysiological mechanisms (mediated by long-lasting changes in gene expression and their downstream consequences) as a result of repeated occurrences of seizures. In this seizure model, this pattern can be inhibited and drug responsitvity can be temporarily reinstated by several manipulations, including lowering illness drive (decreasing the stimulation current), increasing drug dosage, switching to a new drug that does not show crosstolerance to the original medication, or temporarily discontinuing treatment, allowing the illness to re-emerge in an unmedicated animal. Each of these variables is discussed in relation to the potential relevance to the emergence, progression, and suppression of individual patterns of episodic cyclicity in the recurrent affective disorders. A variety of clinical studies are outlined that specifically test the hypothesis derived from this formulation. Data from animal studies suggest that illness cyclicity can develop from the relative ratio between primary pathological processes and secondary endogenous adaptation (assisted by exogenous medications). If this proposition is verified, it further suggests that illness cyclicity is inherent to the neurobiological processes of episode emergence and amelioration, and one does not need to postulate a separate defect in the biological clock. The interventions may be optimal in order to prevent illness emergence and progression and its associated accumulating neurobiological vulnerability factors.

40. Post, R.M. & Weiss, S. B., (1995). F.E. Bloom (Ed.), & D.J. Kupfer (Ed.), *Psychopharmacology: The Fourth Generation of Progress.* (pp 1155-69). Raven Press,. Ltd., New York. **See Book**

From the introduction: In 1921, Kraepelin not only differentiated manic-depressive illness from schizophrenia, but he crystallized the critical observation on the longitudinal development of the illness based on his systematic [human] patient records and life-chart methodology. He described the pleomorphic ["more than one distinct form"] aspects of its clinical presentation and the tremendous variability in its clinical course. At the same time, he abstracted the general principle that patients often undergo a pattern of cycle acceleration with longer intervals occurring between the first and second episodes than those occurring later in the illness do. He also noted a progression from precipitated to autonomous episodes, such that psychosocial stresses (particularly loss or the threat of loss) appeared to be implicated in initial episodes but not in subsequent episodes, which occur more spontaneously, that is, without apparent external precipitating factors. It is against this backdrop of a potentially progressive and evolving illness that issues of treatment resistance should be considered. In the ensuing decades, these initial clinical observations have been documented and redocumented in more formal clinical studies. In systematic studies examining the issue of cycle acceleration, the general pattern of decreasing duration of well intervals as a function of successive episodes has been supported in virtually every study. **From THE Section Called,** *Kindling As A Model For Illness Evolution And Transition To Autonomy.* In contrast to the behavioral sensitization described above [cocaine sensitization in rats], which directly models many aspects of [human] mood illness (particularly euphoric and dysphoric [sad] manias), [electrical] kindling [in rats] is a nonhomologous [does not exhibit a biologically similar] model for [human] mood illness evolution. Increased behavioral reactivity [in electrically stimulated rats] is measured with a seizure endpoint, and none of the behaviors in [electrical] kindling evolution [in rats] are similar to those observed in [human] patients with bipolar illness. Thus, although we might consider how various aspects of bipolar illness undergo kindling-like transitions, it must be restated that kindling is only a conceptual bridge that might help describe the kinds of neurobiological processes, and their spatial and temporal evolution, in the brain that could be associated with the progression of a disorder. Given these caveats, which violate most of the traditional principles of animal modeling of mood disorders, why discuss kindling as a potentially useful model in this context at all? In [electrical] kindling, there is (a) increased behavioral responsivity to the same stimulation over time and (b) a progression to spontaneity following sufficient numbers of triggered kindled seizures. These syndrome characteristics are paralleled in vastly different time domains in some patients with mood disorders. **From the section,** ***Stress And Episode Sensitization In The Recurrent Mood Disorders:*** "The postulate is that, as in sensitization and kindling, appropriate psychosocial stressors may, through their impact on IEGs and late effector genes, reach a threshold for inducing full-blown episodes of affective illness...These observations also imply that another phenomenon is occurring simultaneously–that of episode sensitization. That is, it is the recurrence of sufficient numbers of triggered affective episodes themselves (similar to that observed with amygdala-kindled seizures) that not only leaves the organism progressively more vulnerable to subsequent episodes, but eventually results in the occurrence of episodes in the absence of exogenous triggers. **From the *Conclusion*:** In the course of affective evolution, we have postulated that, based on alterations in experience-induced gene expression, there is sensitization both to stressors and to episodes themselves. In the kindling process, each apparently similar and behaviorally stereotyped occurrence of a seizure episode appears, nonetheless, to propel the process gradually toward autonomy (i.e., the spontaneous occurrence of seizures with their differential anatomy and pharmacology). If a similar phenomenon were found to occur in the different neural systems implicated in the mood disorders, then one would postulate not only that repeated episodes may propel the illness toward autonomy, but that a differential pharmacology may also exist as a function of stage-of-illness evolution.

41. Post, R.M.; Weiss, S.B.; & Leverich, G.S., (1994). Recurrent affective disorder: Roots in developmental neurobiology and illness progression based on changes in gene expression. *Development and Psychopathology,* 6, 4: 81-813.

Abstract: Electrophysiological kindling and behavioral sensitization to psychomotor stimulants and stress provide paradigms for understanding how repeated acute events can leave neurobiological residues in gene expression. In kindling, a complex spatiotemporal cascade of events occurs, including induction of immediate early and late effector genes. Behavioral sensitization to psychomotor stimulants and stress induces related, but different cascades of effects on the expression of these genes. If these types of alterations are put into a developmental context, this would provide a paradigm for understanding how early life events could exert profound and behaviorally relevant biochemical and microstructural effects on the CNS of the developing organism. The conceptual overview offered by the sensitization and kindling models suggests that environmentally triggered neurobiological processes do not form a single or static residue. ((c) 1997 APA/PsycINFO, all rights reserved).

42. Post, R.M. & Silberstein, S.D., (1994). Shared mechanisms in affective illness, epilepsy, and migraine. *Neurology, 44, 10, [Suppl. 7]:* S37-S47.

Abstract: For a specific subgroup of patients with migraine or affective illness who experience illness progression and drug tolerance, the amygdala kindling paradigm can be a useful, but nonhomologous, model. Although these patients do not have a seizure or seizure-like disorder, kindling has been used to examine the types of memory-like mechanisms that could underlie syndrome evolution in both migraine and affective illness. While the precipitants, symptomatology, duration of attack, and aura symptoms differ among epilepsy, migraine and affective disorders, all are paroxysmal dysregulations that partially share effective drug treatment. The principles of seizure progression presented here may apply to affective and migraine patients whose episodes progress from isolated and intermittent to more chronic or daily. These patients may also develop tolerance to long-term prophylactic treatments.

43. Post, R.M.; Ketter, T.A.; Pazzaglia, P.J.; Denicoff, K; Marangell, L.; George, M.S, (1994). Nolen, W.A. (Ed); Zohar, J. (Ed); et.al. *Refractory depression: Current strategies and future directions*, (pp 97-114). Chichester, England UK: John Wiley & Sons. xvi, 235 pp. **SEE BOOK**

Abstract: (From the preface): Review the use of anticonvulsants, carbamazepine and valproate, in lithium-refractory patients. (From the chapter): Carbamazepine / contingent tolerance: Clinical and theoretical implications / valproate and other anticonvulsant agents / possible predictors of clinical response / sensitization and kindling models: Implications for treatment with anticonvulsants. ((c) 1997 APA/PsycINFO, all rights reserved).

44. Post, R.M. (1994). Mechanisms underlying the evolution of affective disorders: Implications for long-term treatment. Grunhaus, L. (Ed.); Greden, J.F. (Ed.); et.al. Severe depressive disorders. *Progress in psychiatry, No. 44.* (pp. 23-65). Washington D.C. USA: American Psychiatric Press, Inc. xxiii, 361 pp. **SEE BOOK**

Abstract: (From the preface): Explains in detail the potential interactions between genetics, environment, cell biology and mood disorders. (From the chapter): Raises the subject of…potential risks of episode recurrence based on failure to institute and maintain prophylaxis / suggests the possibility that the evolution of the illness itself may change in a more malignant direction following repeated episode occurrence / this might include not only cycle acceleration, but also the potential for drug refractoriness / the discussion of illness progression is presented with the backdrop that experience of acute stressors, and even episodes of affective illness themselves, may leave behind "memory traces" at the level of altered gene expression that make The patient more vulnerable to subsequent recurrences /// the transition from precipitated to spontaneous episodes / potential mechanisms underlying stress sensitization: Impact on gene expression / effects of kindling on gene transcription: A spatiotemporal approach to the kindled memory trace / implications of sensitization and kindling for the progressive evolution of affective illness / implications for therapeutics / review of evidence of the efficacy of prophylaxis in unipolar depression / impediments to long-term treatment: The myth of mental illness / patient and public information: Overcoming stigma and ignorance / recommendations for early prophylaxis. ((c) 1997 APA/PsycINFO, all rights reserved).

45. Post, R.M. (1992). Transduction of psychosocial stress into the neurobiology of recurrent affective disorder. *American Journal of Psychiatry*, *149, 8:* 99-1010.

Abstract: Early clinical observations and recent systematic studies overwhelmingly document a greater role for psychosocial stressor in association with the first episode of major affective disorder than with subsequent episodes. The author postulates that both sensitization to stressors and episode sensitization occurs and become encoded at the level of gene expression. In particular, stressors and the biochemical concomitants of the episodes themselves can induce the proto-oncogene c-fos and related transcription factors, which then affect the expression of transmitters, receptors and neuropeptides that alter responsivity in a long-lasting fashion. Thus, both stressors and episodes may leave residual traces and vulnerabilities to further occurrences of affective illness. These data and concepts suggest that the biochemical and anatomical substrates underlying the affective disorders evolve over time as a function of recurrences, as does pharmacological responsivity. This formulation highlights the critical importance of early intervention in the illness in order to prevent malignant transformation to rapid cycling, spontaneous episodes, and refractoriness to drug treatment.

46. Post, R.M.; Altshuler, L.L.; Ketter, T.A.; Denicoff, K.; Weiss, S.R.B., (1991). Antiepileptic drugs in affective illness: Clinical and theoretical implications. Smith, D.B. (Ed.); Treiman, D.M. (Ed.); et.al., Neurobehavioral problems in epilepsy. *Advances in neurology 55,* (pp. 239-277). New York, NY, USA: Raven Press, Publishers. xx, 485 pp. **See Book.**

Abstract: (From the chapter): Briefly reviews the evidence for the efficacy of a variety of anticonvulsant modalities in the acute and prophylactic treatment of manic-depressive illness /// start with a consideration of electroconvulsive therapy as the best documented and most efficacious treatment of acute depressive episodes and include it under the rubric of an anticonvulsant since recent data suggest that it is, in fact, a potent anticonvulsant modality in both humans and experimental animals /// the question is raised and discussed as to whether the anticonvulsant properties of these agents are, in fact, related to their psychotropic effects in manic-depressive patients / this issue obviously becomes crucial when considering mechanisms of action of the anticonvulsants, both in seizure disorders and in affective disorders /// some evidence suggests that temporal factors such as the time course of onset of efficacy may be different in seizure and affective disorders, suggesting that different mechanisms are involved /// evidence is addressed on the issue of whether limbic sites of action of the anticonvulsants are, in fact, related to their positive effects in manic-depressive illness /// finally, the kindling analogy for the evolution of symptoms in the course of affective illness is discussed in the context of its potential derivative theoretical implications for a differential pharmacotherapy as a function of illness, since this analogy may help in elucidation of the phenomenon of conditioned tolerance. ((c) 1997 APA/PsycINFO, all rights reserved).

47. Post, R.M.; Weiss, S., (1990). Sensitization, kindling, and carbamazepine: An update on their implications for the course of affective illness. *Pharmacopsychiatry 25, 1:* 41-43.

Abstract: Discusses 2 preclinical models (behavioral sensitization to psychomotor stimulants and electrophysiological kindling) for conceptualizing mechanisms underlying the progressive and evolving aspects of manic-depressive illness and examines the acute and long-term effectiveness of the anticonvulsant carbamazepine. Peripheral-type and alpha-2 adrenergic benzodiazepine receptors and stabilization of type-2 sodium channels may be involved in the anticonvulsant effects of carbamazepine. Gamma-aminobutyric acid-sub(B) (GABA-sub(B)) mechanisms are thought to be related to the antinociceptive, but not the anticonvulsant or psychotropic, effects of carbamazepine. Many neurotransmitters remain candidates for the pychotropic effects. An animal model requiring chronic administration of carbamazepine to show efficacy is reported. (German abvstract) ((c) 1009 APA/PsycINFO, all rights reserved).

48. Post, R.M., (1990). Prophylaxis of bipolar affective disorders. *International Review of Psychiatry, 2, 3-4:* 277-320

Abstract: Discusses the prophylaxis (absence of episodes) of bipolar disorders, stressing the importance of life charting methodology in assessing course of illness and response to pharmacologic interventions. Preliminary evidence suggests that some variables associated with lithium nonresponse may be associated with a good response to carbamazepine or valproate (either alone or in combination with lithium). Data suggest that the use of thyroid hormones and calcium channel blockers may be of clinical utility with the refractory bipolar patient. Two preclinical models (i.e., behavioral sensitization to psychomotor stimulants and electrophysiological kindling) may have heuristic value in assessing principles underlying the progressive evolution of psychopathological and neuropathological syndromes. ((c) 1997 APA/PsycINFO, all rights reserved).

49. Post, R.M.; Weiss, S.R.B.; Clark, M.; Nakajima, T.; Pert, A., (1990). Amygdala versus local anesthetic kindling: Differential anatomy, pharmacology, and clinical implications. Wada, J.A. (Ed.); et.al., Kindling 4. *Advances in behavioral biology 37*, (pp.357-370). New York, NY, USA: Plenum Press. xiii, 477 pp. **SEE BOOK**

Abstract*:* (From the chapter): focuses on one specific type of pharmacological kindling; i.e., that associated with local anesthetic administration /// electrical kindling of the amygdala and local anesthetic kindling achieved with lidocaine and cocaine are compared and contrasted /// while the emphasis is on the differential efficacy of pharmacological interventions in these two types of kindling, anatomical, physiological, and behavioral data are also briefly considered /// a striking double dissociation is observed in that the same anticonvulsant, carbamazepine, which is potent in blocking completed amygdala-kindled seizures, but not their development, is highly effective in blocking the development of local-anesthetic seizures, but their complete variety. ((c) 1997 APA/PsycINFO, all rights reserved).

50. Post, R.M. (1989). Introduction: Emerging perspectives on valproate in affective disorders. *Journal of Clinical Psychiatry 50, [3 Suppl.]*: 3-9

Abstract: The anticonvulsants, especially carbamazepine and valproate, offer new clinical and theoretical perspectives in the treatment of lithium-refractory bipolar disorders. They appear effective in a group of patients who often respond poorly to lithium, that is, those with rapid cycling illness. Given that these drugs have different profiles of clinical antiepileptic activity and different biochemical mechanisms of action, it is not unexpected that preliminary evidence indicates that some affectively ill patients may selectively respond to one agent, but not to the other. It remains to be determined whether common mechanisms underlie the anticonvulsant and pychotropic effects and whether "limbic" actions are important to their properties in affective illness. The potential role of valproate in acute and long-term treatment of bipolar illness deserves further controlled evaluation given the preliminary data summarized in the series of papers in this volume.

51. Post, R.M.; Weiss, S., (1989). Kindling and manic-depressive illness. Bolwig, T.G. (Ed); Trimble, M.R. (Ed); et.al. *The clinical relevance of kindling,* (pp. 209-230). Chichester, England UK: John Wiley & Sons. xi, 302 pp. **SEE BOOK**

Abstract: (From the chapter): we hope to use the kindling analogy to help us focus on the longitudinal course of manic-depressive illness and raise a series of questions based on preclinical data that deserve careful clinical and theoretical investigation /// also attempt to distinguish the phenomenon of behavioral sensitization to psychomotor stimulants from that of electrophysiological kindling /// cocaine-induced behavioral sensitization / electrical and pharmacological kindling / contingent inefficacy and contingent tolerance ((c) 1997 APA/PsycINFO, all rights reserved).

52. Post, R.M.; Uhde, T.W.; Putnam, F.W.; Ballenger, J.C.; and Berrettini, W.H. (1982). Kindling and carbamazepine in affective illness. *The Journal of Nervous and Mental Disease, 170,12:* 17-731.

Abstract: Kindling represents a process in which increasing behavioral and convulsive responses occur to repetition of the same stimulus over time. Increased behavioral response can also occur to repetition of the same dose of psychomotor stimulant or dopamine agonist, i.e., behavioral sensitization. These two models, which may have important implications for the progressive development of psychopathology in a variety of neuropsychiatric syndromes, are reviewed. Carbamazepine, a drug of choice in treatment of temporal lobe and limbic seizures, and effective in inhibiting kindling, has been used as a treatment of primary and secondary affective illness. The efficacy of carbamazepine in affective illness and its clinical and theoretical implications are discussed.

53. Rosen, J.B. & Schulkin, Jay (1998). From Normal Fear to Pathological Anxiety. *Psychological Review, 105*, 2: 325-350.

Abstract: In this article, the authors address how pathological anxiety may develop from adaptive fear states. Fear responses (e.g., freezing, startle, heart rate and blood pressure changes, and increased vigilance) are functionally adaptive behavioral and perceptual responses elicited during danger to facilitate appropriate defensive responses that can reduce danger or injury (e.g., escape and avoidance). Fear is a central motive state of action tendencies subserved by fear circuits, with the amygdala playing a central role. Pathological anxiety is conceptualized as an exaggerated fear state in which hyperexcitability of fear circuits that include the amygdala and extended amygdala (i.e., bed nucleus of the stria terminalis) is expressed as hypervigilance and increased behavioral responsivity to fearful stimuli. Reduced thresholds for activation and hyperexcitability in fear circuits develop through sensitization, or **kindling-like**, processes that involve neuropeptides, hormones, and other proteins. Hyperexctability in fear circuits is expressed as pathological anxiety that is manifested in the various anxiety disorders.

54. Rush, J.A., M.D. & Suppes, T., M.D., (1998) "What are the new treatments for bipolar disorder?", *The Harvard Mental Health Letter*, January, 74 Fenwood Road, Boston, MA 02115

55. Segal, Z.V.; Williams, J.M.; Teasdale, J.D.; & Gemar, M. (1996). A cognitive science perspective on kindling and episode sensitization in recurrent affective disorder. *Psychological Medicine, 26, 2: 371-380.*

Abstract: Offers a cognitive science analysis of the interaction between psychosocial stress and the neurobiology of affective illness, highlighting major depressive disorder. This analysis builds on observations of R.M. Post (1992) regarding the importance of kindling and sensitization effects in determining activation of neural patterns of information processing being activated in depressed states. As is found in studies of kindling and behavioral sensitization, the likelihood of cognitive patterns being activated is dependent on the frequency of past usage, and increased reliance on these patterns of processing makes it easier for their future activation to occur on the basis of minimal cues. ((c) 1977 APA/PsycINFO, all rights reserved).

56. Sharma, V.; Ainsworth, P.J.; McCabe, S.B., Persand, E.; et., al., (1997). A nongenetic basis of cycle frequency in bipolar disorder: Study of a monozygotic twin pair. *Journal of Psychiatry and Neuroscience 22, 2:* 132-135.

Abstract: Describes the case of a pair of female monozygotic adult twins with bipolar disorder, but with a different course of the illness, including age of onset, sequence of episodes, and cycle length. Twin A initially became depressed at age 13, and over the course of 3 yrs had 2 more episodes. Twin B became depressed at age 17, but was able to cope until the onset of her 1st clinically significant episode 6 mos later. Results show that there is a cycle frequency in bipolar disorder that does not appear to be genetically determined. In this study, the twins were discordant for cycle frequency despite being concordant for bipolar disorder. ((c) 1997 APA/PscyINFO, all rights reserved).

57. Shorter, E., (1997). *A History of Psychiatry*, New York, NY: John Wiley & Sons, Inc.

58. Snyder, K. (1995). New drug indication for mania: First in quarter-century. Drug Topics 139, 13: 38.

Abstract: The Food & Drug Administration has approved an additional treatment indication for mania for Abbott Laboratories' Depakote. The drug, a brand version of divalproex sodium, has been available in the US since 1983 for the treatment of simple and complex absence seizures. The new indication, for patients with bipolar disorder, or manic-depressive illness, represents the first approval of a new drug to treat manic episodes in 25 years. An estimated 2-million-plus Americans suffer from the disorder, yet a third do not seek treatment.

59. Souery, D.; Mendelbaum, K. & Mendlewicz, J. (1994). Genetics and manic-depressive psychosis: review and current findings. *Acta Psychiatr Belg. 94, 3:* 134-150.

Abstract: The present article reviews the basic and recent findings of the genetics in manic-depressive illness. The different molecular genetic techniques that have been applied to this research field are presented. Results of linkage and association studies are discussed in regard to the main limitations of these approaches in psychiatric disorders. On the whole, linkage and association studies contributed to the localization of some potential vulnerability genes for manic-depression on chromosome X and 11, and more recently, 18.

60. Spitzer, R.L., Endicott, J., (1979) *Schedule for Affective Disorders and Schizophrenia, Life-time Version*, Research Assessment and Training Unit, New York State Psychiatric Institute, NYC.

61. No author cited, (1991),Teleconference. Neurobiological Alterations Associated With Post Traumatic Stress Disorder, National Center for PTSD, Clinical Laboratory and Education Division, Department of Veterans Affairs, White River Junction, Vt.

62. http:\www.washingtonpost.com/wp-srv/health/daily/sept99/brain 28.htm

63. Weiss, S.R. & Post, R.M. 1998. Kindling: spearate vs. shared mechanisms in affective disorders and epilepsy. *Neuropsychobiology*, Oct; 38(3): 167-80

Abstract: Kindling is discussed in relation to affective illness as a nonhomologous model, which shares the feature of increasing illness severity and evolution over time following repeated exposures to certain forms of stimulation. This progressive aspect of kindling has proven useful in the study of approaches to pharmacotherapeutics, mechanisms and characteristics of drug tolerance, and, most recently, illness suppression through physiological rather than pharmacological strategies. Each of these themes is described and the mechanisms that have been uncovered using the kindling model are discussed in relation to how similar principles might apply in affective illness or epilepsy. It is hoped that some of the lessons from the kindling model will provide useful and novel insights into aspects of treatment and mechanisms of psychiatric and neurologic illnesses.

64. Wender, P.H. & Klein, D.F., (1981), *Mind, Mood, and Medicine.* New York, N.Y., Farrar, Straus, Giroux.

65. WWWebster Dictionary copyright © 2000 by Merriam-Webster, Incorporated